# THE RACE TO MANUFACTURE COVID-19 VACCINES
## EMERGING VACCINE TECHNOLOGIES

NOVEMBER 2023

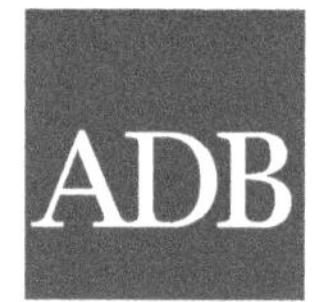

ASIAN DEVELOPMENT BANK

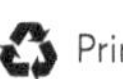 Printed on recycled paper

# Contents

# Tables and Figure

**Tables**



**Figure**

# Abbreviations

| | | |
|---|---|---|
| ADB | – | Asian Development Bank |
| DMC | – | developing member country |
| COVID-19 | – | coronavirus disease |
| DNA | – | deoxyribonucleic acid |
| EUA | – | emergency use authorization |
| EUL | – | emergency use listing |
| GMP | – | good manufacturing practice |
| LMICs | – | low- and middle-income countries |
| MHRA | – | Medicines and Healthcare Products Regulatory Agency (United Kingdom) |
| mRNA | – | messenger ribonucleic acid |
| nAb | – | neutralizing antibody |
| RBD | – | receptor binding domain |
| RSV | – | respiratory syncytial virus |
| S-2P | – | recombinant spike protein |
| TGA | – | Therapeutic Goods Administration |
| US FDA | – | United States Food and Drug Administration |

## WEIGHTS AND MEASURES

| | | |
|---|---|---|
| g | – | gram |
| l | – | liter |
| ml | – | milliliter |

# I.  Introduction

The global outbreak of the coronavirus disease (COVID-19) in 2020 was the driver for Australia's Therapeutic Goods Administration (TGA) to conduct horizon scanning for new vaccines and new vaccine production technologies.

This paper summarizes a selection of the products and technologies identified during this horizon scanning to inform national COVID-19 responses of Asian Development Bank (ADB) developing member countries (DMCs), as well as to inform initiatives to strengthen vaccine manufacturing in Asia and the Pacific. For example, DMCs may use this information to assist with investment decisions related to vaccine procurement and manufacturing.

The 16 companies included in this paper were identified by the TGA as developing emerging vaccine technologies (Table 1). All companies signed confidential disclosure agreements with TGA during 2021–2022 to work with ADB to assist DMCs in Asia and the Pacific. Some companies are employing established technological platforms adapted to new pathogens like the severe acute respiratory syndrome coronavirus 2 (SARS-CoV-2), the causative agent of COVID-19, while others are developing novel technologies.

## Table 1: List of Vaccines and Products by Manufacturer

| Company | Vaccine/Product Type | Vaccine Subtype |
|---|---|---|
| Arcturus Therapeutics | Component viral | Ribonucelic acid |
| Baiya Phytopharm | Component viral | Protein subunit |
| Beijing Wantai Biological Pharmacy Enterprise | Component viral | Nonreplicating viral vector |
| Biological E. Limited | Component viral | Protein subunit |
| CanSino Biologics, Inc. | Component viral | Nonreplicating viral vector |
| Codagenix | Whole virus | Live-attenuated |
| HDT Bio | Component viral | Ribonucelic acid |
| Medigen Vaccine Biologics Corp | Component viral | Protein subunit |
| Nanogen Pharmaceutical Biotechnology | Component viral | Protein subunit |
| Providence Therapeutics | Component viral | Ribonucelic acid |
| Raphael Labs | Prophylactic spray | |
| Sanofi | Component viral | Protein subunit |
| Shionogi | Component viral | Protein subunit |
| Valneva | Whole virus | Inactivated |
| Vaxxas | Skin patch | |
| Vaxxinity | Component viral | Protein subunit |

Source: Asian Development Bank.

# II.  Overview of Vaccine Platforms

There are different types of COVID-19 vaccines made from part or all of the SARS-CoV-2 virus. All vaccines aim to stimulate the body's immune system, so that if a vaccinated person encounters the COVID-19 virus, the vaccine can remove it from the body (Figure).

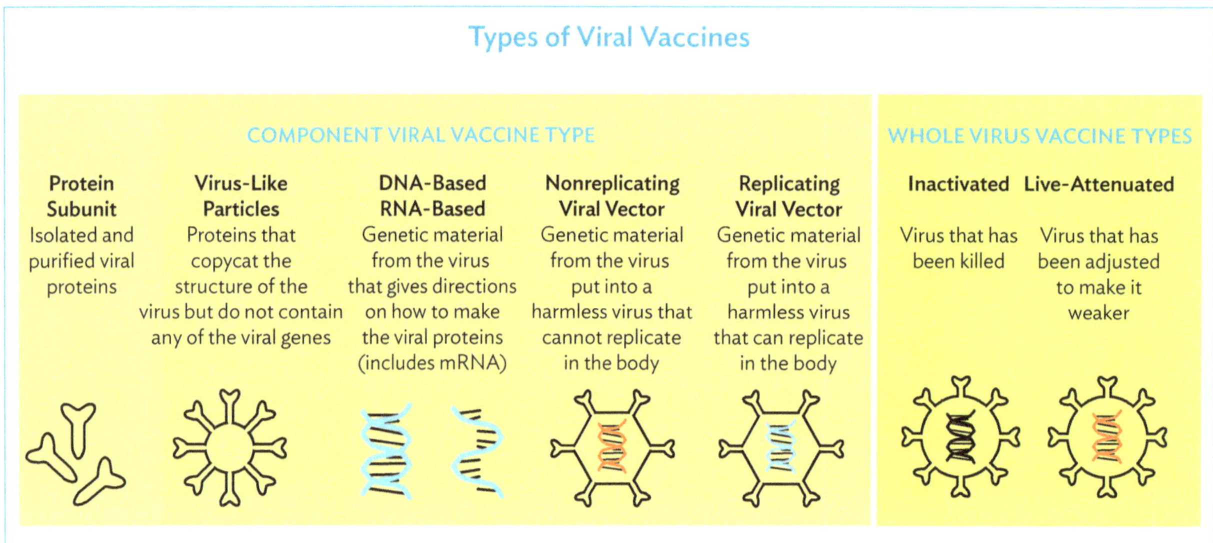



COVID-19 = coronavirus disease, DNA = deoxyribonucleic acid, mRNA = messenger ribonucleic acid, RNA = ribonucleic acid.

Source: Adapted from COVID-19 Vaccine Tracker. https://covid19.trackvaccines.org/types-of-vaccines/ (accessed 1 September 2023).

# III. Vaccine Briefs

Each of the 16 manufacturer summaries here includes, where relevant, the following content:

(i)     background information about the manufacturer;
(ii)    a description of the vaccine platforms and/or technologies employed by the manufacturer;
(iii)   details of COVID-19 vaccine(s) developed;
(iv)    details of vaccine pipeline; and
(v)     existing partnerships and approach to working with ADB's DMCs or low- and middle-income countries (LMICs).

## A. Arcturus Therapeutics (United States)

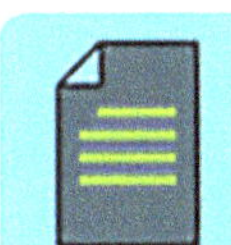

### 1. Background

Arcturus Therapeutics is a late-stage clinical messenger ribonucleic acid (mRNA) and deoxyribonucleic acid (DNA) medicines and vaccines company. It was founded in 2013 and is based in the United States (US). The company has set its sights on producing vaccines for communicable diseases and therapeutics for rare respiratory diseases.

### 2. Vaccine Platform and Technologies

#### (i) LUNAR Delivery System

LUNAR is a proprietary lipid-mediated nucleic acid delivery system developed by Arcturus that aims to improve the delivery, tolerance, and safety of nucleic acid-based medicines (Mucker et al. 2020). The LUNAR system encapsulates and delivers therapeutic nucleic acids to specific cells by endocytosis (Ramaswamy  et al. 2017; Perez-Garcia et al. 2022; Diaz-Trelles et al. 2022): particles fuse to the membrane of the cell and then bring the mRNA or DNA inside the cell. This corrects the genetic defect and allows the cell to produce healthy proteins.

The lipids do not accumulate inside the cell allowing for repeated dosing. Use of LUNAR may require a smaller amount of active pharmaceutical ingredient for therapeutic effects, potentially reducing the risk of adverse events. LUNAR can be administered by multiple routes—intravenous, intramuscular, inhaled, nebulized, subretinal, and intravitreal—and can deliver mixtures of different mRNAs as a single drug product. The lipids have been tailored to be highly efficient at encapsulating mRNA and DNA, which also reduces manufacturing costs.

## (ii)  STARR Delivery System

The STARR delivery system specifically combines LUNAR with self-replicating RNA (srRNA). This can be used for prophylactic vaccines that stimulate antigen expression within host cells, leading to long-term protective immunity against selected infections. In addition, srRNA-based vaccines require lower doses than non-srRNA-based vaccines, and production is fast and simple (Lundstrom et al. 2021).

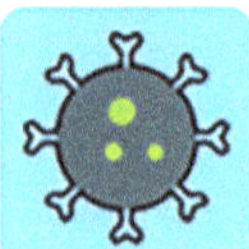

## 3.  COVID-19 Vaccine

The COVID-19 vaccine booster candidate, ARCT-154, was developed using the STARR technology and may offer advantages including low-dose (5 micrograms), lyophilized formulation, acceptable vaccine efficacy, durability, and safety profile, as well as rapid global scale-up, and improved supply chain and distribution. The vaccine also does not use any adjuvants or viral vectors.

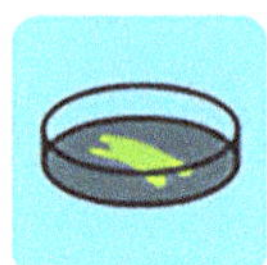

## 4.  Vaccine Pipeline

Arcturus is developing numerous mRNA vaccine candidates to prevent COVID-19 (Alwis et al. 2021) and influenza infections.

The company is also developing an mRNA medicine for ornithine transcarbamylase (OTC) deficiency, the most common urea cycle disorder in humans (Yu et al. 2022). OTC deficiency causes ammonia to build up in the blood.  Without a liver transplantation, currently the only cure for OTC deficiency, the high levels of ammonia can lead to neurological damage, coma, and death.

In addition, Arcturus is collaborating with the Cystic Fibrosis Foundation in the US to develop an mRNA medicine (Pei et al. 2022). Over time, cystic fibrosis leads to irreversible damage to the respiratory tract and gut. While treatments have improved, people with cystic fibrosis still typically die in their mid-40s (Table 2).

### Table 2: Vaccine Pipeline for Arcturus Therapeutics

| Vaccine Name | Indication Group | Development Stage | | | | | |
| --- | --- | --- | --- | --- | --- | --- | --- |
| | | Discovery | Preclinical | Phase 1 | Phase 2 | Phase 3 | Registration |
| LUNAR-COV19 ARCT-154 as Booster Vaccine | COVID-19 | | | | | | |
| LUNAR-COV19 ARCT-154 as Primary Vaccine | COVID-19 | | | | | | |
| LUNAR FLU | Influenza | | | | | | |
| LUNAR-OTC ARCT-810 | OTC Deficiency | | | | | | |
| LUNAR-CF ARCT-032 | Cystic Fibrosis | | | | | | |

COVID-19 = coronavirus disease, OTC = over-the-counter.

Source: Arcturus.

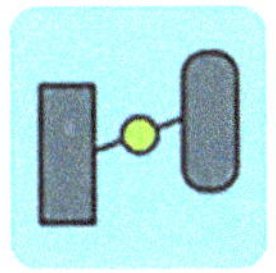

## 5. Partnerships and/or Approach to Working with Low- and Middle-Income Countries

Arcturus has partnered with several industry leaders to bolster its preclinical drug development pipeline.

External development partners (Table 3) include CureVac AG; Janssen Pharmaceuticals, Inc. (Johnson & Johnson); Synthetic Genomics Inc.; Takeda Pharmaceutical Company Limited; and Ultragenyx Pharmaceutical Inc. Treatments for a range of gastrointestinal disorders have been developed including glycogen storage disease type III, Hepatitis B virus infection, and nonalcoholic steatohepatitis (NASH).

### Table 3: Arcturus Therapeutics' Partnerships

| Program | Partner | Indication | Stage |
|---|---|---|---|
| LUNAR-GSDIII | Ultragenyx Pharmaceutical Inc. | Glycogen Storage Disease Type III | Phase 1/2 |
| LUNAR-RARE | Ultragenyx Pharmaceutical Inc. | N/A | Preclinical |
| LUNAR-HBV | Johnson & Johnson | HBV | Preclinical |
| LUNAR-NASH | Takeda Pharmaceutical Company Limited | NASH | Preclinical |

HBV = Hepatitis B virus, NASH = nonalcoholic steatohepatitis.
Source: Arcturus.

In 2020, Arcturus and Duke-NUS Medical School used the STARR technology to produce a COVID-19 vaccine for the Singapore Economic Development Board. In 2021, Arcturus announced an agreement with Vingroup, the largest conglomerate in Viet Nam, focusing on technology, health care, industry, real estate development, retail, and hospitality. This agreement aims to build a manufacturing plant in Viet Nam for COVID-19 vaccines for domestic use. Under the agreement, Vinbiotech will build the manufacturing facility while Arcturus will provide access to proprietary technologies and processes to manufacture COVID-19 vaccines. The license and technology transfer applies to drug product manufacturing. Other global manufacturing partners include Aldevron (US), Catalent (US), Recipharm (Germany), Polymun Scientific (Austria), and ARCALIS (Japan).

In November 2022, Arcturus signed a major licensing deal (Reuters 2022) with Australian vaccine manufacturer CSL, which gives CSL's vaccine arm, CSL Seqirus, an (i) exclusive license to Arcturus's next-generation mRNA technology for medical products for respiratory diseases, including COVID-19 and influenza; and (ii) nonexclusive rights to develop vaccines and therapeutics that can address multiple diseases of pandemic potential.

# B. Baiya Phytopharm (Thailand)

## 1. Background

Founded in 2018 as a startup company within the Chulalongkorn University Faculty of Pharmaceutical Sciences in Bangkok, Thailand, Baiya Phytopharm's vaccine technology aspires to replace biotech's fermenter of animal cells with plant-based biologics (Shanmugaraj et al. 2021). The company claims this platform may dramatically accelerate biopharmaceutical manufacturing—products may be produced in weeks—and reduce costs for research and development (R&D).

Baiya Phytopharm has a current good manufacturing practice (GMP) facility of 1,200 square meters in Bangkok, licensed for manufacturing clinical trial products by the Food and Drug Administration of Thailand. The company claims this facility can produce clinical materials of plant-produced protein to supply up to 60 million vaccine doses yearly. Baiya Phytopharm's suite of products helps move Thailand toward sustainability in health care and vaccine production and further develops the nation's pharmaceutical industry.

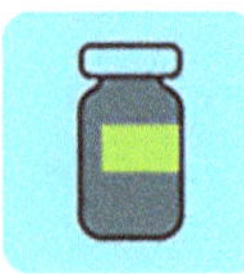

### 2.  Vaccine Platform and Technologies

Baiya Phytopharm's recombinant protein expression system uses the leaves of an Australian heirloom tobacco plant, *Nicotiana benthamiana*, as the platform for transient expression. This plant is said to offer advantages over other plant expression systems: easy, fast, low-cost, and produces high yields of recombinant proteins.

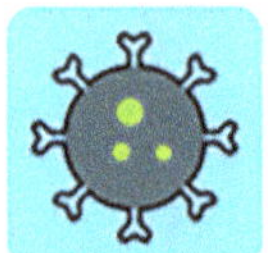

### 3.  COVID-19 Vaccines

Baiya Phytopharm has examined the use of the plant-produced receptor-binding domain (RBD) of the SARS-CoV-2 virus as a subunit COVID-19 vaccine, Baiya SARS-CoV-2 Vax 1. The RBD was joined with an Fc fragment of human IgG1 and transiently expressed in *Nicotiana benthamiana by agro-infiltration* (Shanmugaraj et al. 2022). In one study (Siriwattananon et al. 2021), two intramuscular injections of the RBD-Fc protein (using alum as an adjuvant) were administered in mice, monkeys, and rats 3 weeks apart on days 0 and 21. Inoculation elicited high neutralization titers, reduced the level of virus in the brain and lungs, protected all the animals against challenge with SARS-CoV-2, and induced cell-mediated and humoral immune responses, as well as vaccine-specific T-cell responses.

The animals in the study remained healthy, and no pathological changes related to the vaccine were found. Further, the vaccine was tolerated at the highest concentrations tested. Another study of monkeys (Khorattanakulchai et al. 2022a) immunized with three intramuscular doses of the vaccine found that their sera induced a neutralizing antibody (nAb) response against five SARS-CoV-2 variants (Alpha, Beta, Gamma, Delta, Omicron). The Delta and Epsilon RBD-Fc-based vaccines also displayed cross-reactive immunogenicity in monkeys, raising the prospect that this plant-derived vaccine could be used after primary vaccination to boost broadly neutralizing antibodies (Khorattanakulchai et al. 2022b). A separate study demonstrated immunogenicity in mice (Panapitakkul et al. 2022).

These results show promise that the plant-produced SARS-CoV-2 RBD may be used as an effective COVID-19 vaccine candidate. Human clinical trials are ongoing.

Baiya Phytopharm has also developed a hybrid subunit vaccine that is intended as a multi-strain coronavirus vaccine because it can induce immunity against a broad range of COVID-19 variants. This candidate is currently being tested in nonhuman primate studies.

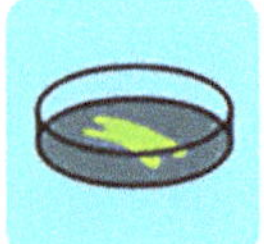

### 4.  Vaccine Pipeline

Baiya Phytopharm is investigating additional biological candidates using their plant-based model as vaccines against infectious diseases and as medicines for cancer. This includes vaccines for infections like COVID-19 and respiratory syncytial virus, as well as cancers of the lung, skin, gastrointestinal system, and breast (Table 4).

Table 4: Vaccine Pipeline for Baiya Phytopharm

| Vaccine Name | Indication Group | Development Stage | | | | | |
|---|---|---|---|---|---|---|---|
| | | Discovery | Preclinical | Phase 1 | Phase 2 | Phase 3 | Commericial |
| BAIYA-SARs-CoV-Vax 1 | COVID-19 | ●━━━━━━━━━━● | | | | | |
| BAIYA-SARs-CoV-Vax 1 | COVID-19 | ●━━━━━━━━━━● | | | | | |
| RSV vaccine | RSV | ●━━━● | | | | | |
| Baiya-CA 001 | Cancer | ●━━━● | | | | | |
| Baiya-CA 002 | Cancer | ●━━━● | | | | | |
| Baiya-CA 003 | Cancer | ●━━━● | | | | | |
| Baiya-CA 004 | Osteoporosis | ●━━━● | | | | | |

COVID-19 = coronavirus disease, RSV = respiratory syncytial virus.

Source: Baiya Phytopharm.

# C. Beijing Wantai Biological Pharmacy Enterprise Co. Ltd. (People's Republic of China)

## 1. Background

Beijing Wantai, established in 1991 in the People's Republic of China (PRC), is a manufacturer of therapeutic goods, including vaccines, infectious disease diagnostic reagents, and medical devices. The company's subsidiary, Innovax, was founded in 2005 to develop vaccines to combat infectious diseases, including Hepatitis E, human papillomavirus (HPV), and COVID-19.

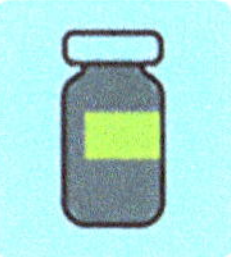

## 2. Vaccine Platform and Technologies

Beijing Wantai's core vaccine platform uses DNA recombinant technology to adopt an established and relatively low-cost *Escherichia coli (E. coli)* expression system. The system was developed in collaboration with the National Institute of Diagnostics and Vaccine Development in Infectious Diseases of Xiamen University.

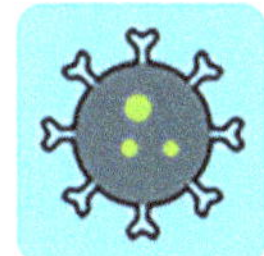

## 3. COVID-19 Vaccine

A live-attenuated influenza virus vector-based SARS-CoV-2 vaccine, dNS1-RBD is delivered by intranasal spray. The vaccine encodes a codon-optimized receptor binding domain (RBD) of the spike (S) protein of the SARS-CoV-2 virus. With nonstructural protein 1 (NS1) of influenza virus deleted, the vector may elicit potent and long-lasting immunity. Preclinical studies of dNS1-RBD suggested that the immune response in the lung was many times stronger than the peripheral blood and that the lungs of hamsters were largely protected after single-dose vaccination and booster vaccination for the most prominent variants, including Omicron (Zhu et al. 2022a; J. Chen et al. 2022). This was despite poor humoral, mucosal, and T-cell immune responses. In addition, dNS1-RBD also provided simultaneous cross-protection against influenza (H1N1 and H5N1 viruses). The vaccine is delivered by syringe, with a special tip designed to produce a mist. Results suggest that the mode of delivering the vaccine into the nose, mouth, and throat may influence the effectiveness of intranasal and inhaled vaccines. Nasal vaccines mimic the way the SARS-CoV-2 virus infects humans and stimulate immunity in the lining of the upper airways.

Data from Phase 3 clinical trials carried out in Colombia, the Philippines, South Africa, and Viet Nam showed that the absolute protective efficacy of the vaccine against COVID-19 within 3 months of vaccination was 55% in those who had not had any previous vaccines; this increased to 82% within 6 months of booster vaccination in the population with vaccination history. The protective efficacy in people aged 60 years or more was similar to people aged 18–59 years. The virus sequenced from the endpoint cases showed that all confirmed cases were Omicron strains, including BA.2 (42%), BA.4 (39%), and BA.5 (18%). This finding indicated that the vaccine had produced effective protection against COVID-19 caused by Omicron infection with a favorable safety profile.

In 2022, dNS1-RBD intranasal vaccine received emergency use authorization (EUA) from the Center for Drug Evaluation of the National Medical Products Administration in the PRC. Beijing Wantai intends to manufacture 200 million doses during the first half of 2023.

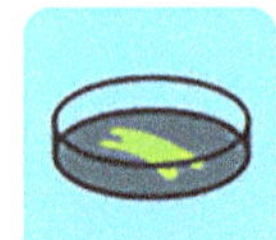

## 4.  Vaccine Pipeline

Numerous vaccines are currently in development and clinical trials (Table 5), including a vaccine against rotavirus, a 20-valent pneumococcal conjugate vaccine (PCV20), and a live varicella vaccine (W. Wang et al. 2022).

Beijing Wantai has three commercially available vaccines:

(i)  **dNS1-RBD.** dNS1-RBD is a live-attenuated influenza virus vector-based SARS-CoV-2 vaccine delivered by intranasal spray. In 2022, it received EUA from the Center for Drug Evaluation of the National Medical Products Administration.

(ii)  **Hecolin.** Hecolin is a Hepatitis E vaccine (Zhu et al. 2010; T. Wu et al. 2012; Zhang et al. 2015). This recombinant virus-like particle vaccine is recommended for those aged 16 years and older who are at high risk of Hepatitis E virus infection. It has marketing authorization in Pakistan and is supplied to Doctors Without Borders (MSF, Médecins Sans Frontières). Registration documents are currently under review in India and Bangladesh.

(iii)  **Cecolin.** Cecolin is a recombinant virus-like particle human papillomavirus (HPV) bivalent (Types 16 and 18) vaccine for preventing cervical cancer (Qiao et al. 2020; Zhao et al. 2022). Cecolin received prequalification from the World Health Organization (WHO) in 2021.[1] Prequalification ensures a vaccine meets international quality, safety, and efficacy standards, and allows the vaccine to enter the global public vaccine market for procurement (Wei et al. 2021), including by United Nations agencies and GAVI, the Vaccine Alliance. Cecolin has received regulatory approval for use in numerous countries, including the PRC, Bangladesh, Morocco, Nepal, and Thailand. Registration documents are currently under review in Cambodia, Democratic Republic of the Congo, Ethiopia, Indonesia, Kazakhstan, Kenya, and Pakistan.

## 5.  Partnerships and/or Approach to Working with Low- and Middle-Income Countries

Beijing Wantai is actively looking for global partnerships, with a focus on low- and middle-income countries (LMICs). The company has signed letters of interest with Indonesia, Pakistan, the Philippines, and Thailand and a memorandum of understanding with Viet Nam. Confidential disclosure agreements have also been signed with 20 companies across 15 countries.

---

[1]  Developing Countries Vaccine Manufacturers Network. New HPV Vaccine from Innovax Receives WHO Prequalification. https://dcvmn. org/New-HPV-vaccine-from-Innovax-receives-WHO-Prequalification/.

Table 5: Vaccine Pipeline for Beijing Wantai

| Vaccine Name | Indication Group | Development Stage | | | | | |
|---|---|---|---|---|---|---|---|
| | | Discovery | Preclinical | Phase 1 | Phase 2 | Phase 3 | Registration |
| Cecolin | HPV | ●————————————————————————————► | | | | | ● |
| Hecolin | Hepatitis E | ●————————————————————————————► | | | | | ● |
| Influenza Virus Vector COVID-19 Vaccine for Intranasal Spray | COVID-19 | ●————————————————————————————► | | | | | ● |
| HPV9 Vaccine + JADE | HPV | ●————————————————————————————► | | | | ● | |
| Varicella vaccine | V-Oka | ●————————————————————► | | | ● | | |
| 2nd generation Varicella | VZV-7D | ●————————————————————► | | | ● | | |
| 20-valent PCV | PCV | ●————————► | ● | | | | |
| Recombinant COVID-19 Vaccine | CHO | ●————————► | ● | | | | |
| 20-valent HPV | HPV | ●—● | | | | | |
| Rotavirus Vaccine | Rotavirus | ●—● | | | | | |

CHO = Chinese hamster ovary cells, COVID-19 = coronavirus disease, HPV = human papillomavirus, PCV = pneumococcal conjugate vaccine, VZV-7D = Varicella-zoster virus.

Source: Beijing Wantai.

# D. Biological E. Limited (India)

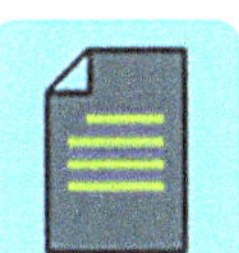

## 1. Background

Biological E. Limited is a biological products company founded in Hyderabad, India, in 1953. The company commenced large-scale production of vaccines against diphtheria, pertussis, and tetanus in 1962. After the construction of a new bacterial, recombinant, and viral vaccine production facility in 2004, Biological E now has four business units: Vaccines and Biologics, Branded Formulations, Specialty Generic Injectables, and Synthetic Biology.

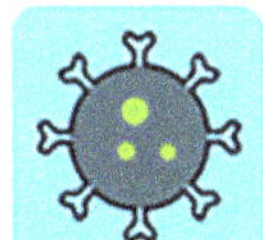

## 2. COVID-19 Vaccine

Biological E has developed the Corbevax protein subunit COVID-19 vaccine. The Drugs Controller General of India issued an EUA for Corbevax in 2021 (*The Times of India* 2021). According to the company, it is in the final stages of a review by WHO for emergency use listing (EUL), based on multiple detailed reviews by the immunization committee of the Strategic Advisory Group of Experts, which has endorsed Corbevax subject to EUL issuance. Corbevax has also been approved for use in Botswana.

The vaccine is based on a platform similar to existing vaccines, such as Hepatitis B. The receptor binding domain (RBD) protein fragment from the S protein of the SARS-CoV-2 virus is used as the antigen. The Center for Vaccine Development at the Texas Children's Hospital in the US developed a recombinant yeast strain that produces the RBD protein, and Biological E licensed this strain from Texas Children's Hospital and Research Technologies Corporation. Biological E scaled up manufacturing processes for RBD production and then developed a COVID-19 vaccine formulation using RBD with adjuvants Alum and CpG1018.

Corbevax has completed five clinical trials. The vaccine demonstrated safety and immunogenicity in children and adolescents (Thuluva et al. 2022b), and in adults following a two-dose primary vaccination series (Pollet et al. 2022; Thuluva 2022a). Corbevax was also examined as a single-dose heterologous booster vaccine in subjects who had received primary vaccination with either a vector-based (AstraZeneca's Vaxzevria and/or Serum Institute of India's Covishield) or inactivated virus-based (Bharat Biotech's Covaxin) vaccine. When administered intramuscularly, Corbevax has been shown to induce significantly elevated nAb titers (Thuluva et al. 2022c). Immunogenicity data for Corbevax suggests a likely vaccine efficiency of more than 90% against the ancestral (Wuhan) strain, and >80% against the Delta strain of SARS-CoV-2 (*India Today* 2022). Vaccination generates a persistent antibody response for more than 6 months.

Biological E has supplied 100 million doses of the Corbevax to the Government of India and accumulated 200 million additional doses (Biological E 2022). Over 73 million doses of Corbevax vaccine have been given to children aged 12–14 years, with 32 million children having received two doses of primary vaccination during the rollout across India. Approximately 7 million doses of Corbevax have also been administered as an adult booster dose in India. The company states it has the capacity to manufacture 100 million doses per month.

Corbevax is supplied to the Government of India at a price of approximately $2.00 per dose and $3.00 per dose in the private market (*Hindustan Times* 2022). It is available in 1-, 10-, and 20-dose presentations with storage requirements of between 2°C and 8°C, which is ordinary refrigeration for vaccine distribution and avoids freezing and thawing. These attributes may improve vaccine access in countries most affected by the COVID-19 pandemic and where new variants are likely to emerge due to low vaccination coverage levels (Solís Arce et al. 2021).

Texas Children's Hospital has licensed the RBD-producing yeast strain to multiple other vaccine producers for the development of COVID-19 vaccines in countries such as Bangladesh and Indonesia, with those vaccines in various stages of development. And because the inventors of Corbevax have not patented the vaccine, anyone with the capacity can reproduce it.

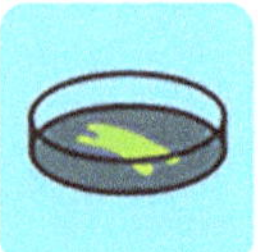

### 3.  Vaccine Pipeline

Biological E currently has eight WHO prequalified vaccines including products for Japanese encephalitis, measles, and rubella; and is expanding its pipeline of biosimilar vaccines.

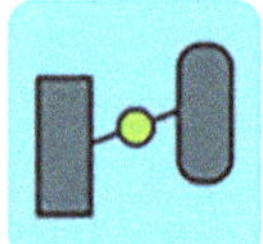

### 4.  Partnerships and/or Approach to Working with Low- and Middle-Income Countries

Biological E has a stated interest in supplying low-cost vaccines to remote parts of the world. This has included commitments to offering its pentavalent vaccine (diphtheria, Hepatitis B, influenza type B, pertussis, tetanus) to GAVI graduated countries with a 30% price reduction.

Biological E has manufacturing facilities in four locations in India that currently manufacture more than 2 million doses of vaccines every day. The company supplies vaccines to global aid organizations and more than 130 countries. Since 2018, it has delivered more than 3 billion doses of vaccines.

# E.  CanSino Biologics, Inc. (People's Republic of China)

### 1.  Background

CanSino was founded in Tianjin in 2009. The company has developed vaccines against numerous diseases, including COVID-19, Ebola, and meningitis. CanSino is concentrating on enhancing the manufacturing of its current portfolio of vaccines, as well as investing in new vaccine candidates.

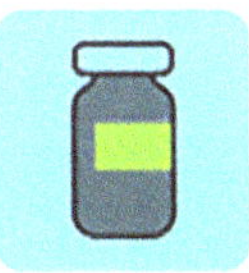

## 2.  Vaccine Platform and Technologies

CanSino has developed several key platform technologies and has licensed new technologies through collaborations with international partners:

(i)    **Viral vector-based technology.** Viral vector-based technology was used to translate the novel Ebola virus vaccine to an approved product in the PRC in 2017 for the national vaccine stockpile. The adenovirus-based vector technology is also used for the tuberculosis booster and other vaccine candidates.

(ii)   **Synthetic vaccine technology.** Synthetic vaccine technology is primarily used to manufacture conjugate vaccines. CanSino produces diphtheria toxoid and tetanus toxoid carrier proteins, as well as CRM197, a carrier protein used in its meningococcal vaccines.

(iii)  **Protein structure design and recombinant technology.** Pneumococcal protein antigens have been developed using a new protein structure design technology. Novel recombinant strains have been used to develop a new-generation pertussis vaccine. CanSino has also developed a proprietary cell line for viral vector vaccines.

(iv)   **mRNA technology.** CanSino's COVID-19 mRNA vaccine (H. Wang et al. 2022), along with other prophylactic virus vaccine candidates, has been developed using this platform.

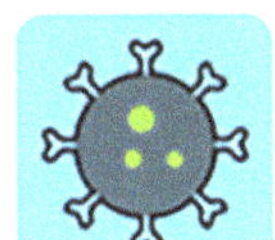

## 3.  COVID-19 Vaccines

(i)        **Recombinant COVID-19 vaccine (adenovirus type 5 vector): Convidecia.** Convidecia uses a third-generation novel coronavirus technology to produce humoral and cellular immunity (Zhu et al. 2020a, 2020b, 2022b; Wu et al. 2021; Halperin et al. 2022; Richardson et al. 2022; Guzmán-López et al. 2022; Li et al. 2022). The vaccine can be stored between 2°C and 8°C. Convidecia has been approved by 11 countries (Argentina, Chile, the PRC, Ecuador, Hungary, Indonesia, Malaysia, Mexico, Moldova, Oman, and Pakistan) and has received EUL from WHO (WHO 2022). CanSino's Tianjin manufacturing facility for Convidecia has been inspected and issued a good manufacturing practice (GMP) certificate by the Hungarian National Institute of Pharmacy and Nutrition, which is a national competent authority in the European Economic Area.

(ii)   **Recombinant COVID-19 vaccine (adenovirus type 5 vector) for inhalation: Convidecia Air.** Convidecia Air is a COVID-19 vaccine for inhalation that induces humoral, cellular, and mucosal immunity. In 2022, it was granted EUA in the PRC and Morocco. It is needle-free, eliminating injection-site reactions, patient fear of needles, and risk of needle-stick injuries to staff, reducing medical waste as well (S. Wu et al. 2021; J. X. Li et al. 2022; Jin et al. 2022; Xu et al. 2022).

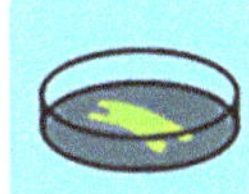

## 4.  Vaccine Pipeline

CanSino's vaccine pipeline comprises 17 vaccines against 12 infectious diseases including Ad5-EBOV, an Ebola vaccine, approved by the PRC in 2017; and two meningococcal vaccines: Group A and Group C Meningococcal Conjugate Vaccine (CRM197) and Group ACYW135 Meningococcal Conjugate Vaccine (CRM197) approved by the PRC in 2021.

CanSino has seven vaccine candidates in clinical trials or undergoing new drug applications, along with five preclinical vaccine candidates under development (Table 6).

## Table 6: Vaccine Pipeline for CanSino

| Vaccine Name | Indication Group | Development Stage | | | | | |
|---|---|---|---|---|---|---|---|
| | | Discovery | Preclinical | Phase 1 | Phase 2 | Phase 3 | Registration |
| Convidecia | COVID-19 | | | | | | ● |
| Adenovirus vector-based Ebola vaccine | Ebola | | | | | | ● |
| Menphecia | Meningococcal | | | | | | ● |
| Menhycia | Meningococcal | | | | | | ● |
| Convidecia Air | COVID-19 | | | | | | ● |
| 13-valent pneumococcal conjugate vaccine | Pneumococcal | | | | | ● | |
| Pneumococcal protein vaccine | Pneumococcal | | | | ● | | |
| Three-component DTaP vaccine for infants | DTaP | | | | | ● | |
| DPT booster vaccine | DPT | | | | | ● | |
| Three-component DTaP vaccine for adolecents and adults | DTaP | | ● | | | | |
| Tuberculosis booster vaccine | Tuberculosis | | | | ● | | |
| mRNA-based COVID-19 vaccines | COVID-19 | | | | ● | | |
| Adenovirus vaccine | N/A | | | ● | | | |
| Combination vaccine | N/A | | | ● | | | |
| Meningococcal B vaccine | Meningococcal | | | ● | | | |
| Shingles vaccine | Herpes | | | ● | | | |
| Polio vaccine | Polio | | | ● | | | |

COVID-19 = coronavirus disease; DPT = diphtheria; DTaP = diphtheria, tetanus, and acellular pertussis vaccine; mRNA = messenger ribonucleic acid; N/A = not applicable.

Source: CanSino.

(i)   **Group A and Group C meningococcal conjugate vaccine (CRM197 vector): Menphecia.** Approved by the PRC, this bivalent meningococcal conjugate vaccine uses the CRM197 vector, a novel carrier protein, which avoids overuse of a single vector. Menphecia provides protection against two serotypes: Group A and Group C.

(ii)  **Group ACYW135 meningococcal conjugate vaccine (CRM197 vector): Menhycia.** Approved by the PRC, Menhycia quadrivalent meningococcal conjugate vaccine provides protection against four types of meningococcal bacteria: types A, C, Y, and W135. Menhycia provides protection for children aged between 3 months and 3 years. Menhycia is the PRC's first, and the world's third, ACYW135 meningococcal conjugate vaccine (Xie et al. 2020, 2021a, 2021b).

(iii) **Recombinant Ebola virus disease vaccine (adenovirus type 5 vector).** This is the third Ebola virus vaccine available globally and the first vaccine approved by an Asian country, the PRC (Zhu et al. 2015, 2017; J.X. Li et al. 2017; Y. Li et al. 2018).

## 5. Partnerships and/or Approach to Working with Low- and Middle-Income Countries

In 2021, CanSino partnered with a Mexican company to establish its first overseas fill-and-finish production line for vaccines. Also in 2021, Pakistan's National Institute of Health commenced a local fill-and-finish line for the Convidecia COVID-19 vaccine, and CanSino helped Malaysia set up a local fill-and-finish line for Convidecia through technology transfer. These production lines enable efficient supply, improving the accessibility and affordability of vaccines in developing countries. CanSino states it is committed to continuing work with countries, particularly in Asia, to facilitate an equitable global distribution of vaccines.

# F. Codagenix (United States)

## 1. Background

Codagenix is a clinical-stage US biotechnology company centered on developing new live vaccines and viral therapeutics. The company combines codon deoptimization and live-attenuated virus design to produce synthetic products that address communicable diseases and cancers in both people and animals.

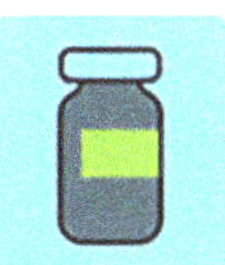

## 2. Vaccine Platform and Technologies

Codagenix's codon deoptimized live-attenuated vaccine candidates may be able to deliver the benefits of live vaccines in short timelines and with robust genetic stability (Coleman et al. 2008). The company uses established manufacturing techniques for its vaccine and therapeutics. Live-attenuated viruses can be produced in cell culture and stored in conventional refrigeration between 2°C and 8°C. These vaccines also have dose-sparing potential to accelerate their distribution in emergency situations (Roozen et al. 2022).

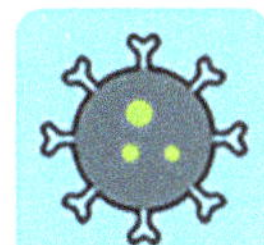

## 3. COVID-19 Vaccines

(i)   **CoviLiv.** CoviLiv (Codagenix 2022b) is a live-attenuated vaccine for prevention of severe COVID-19 (Y. Wang et al. 2021).

(ii)  **Intranasal vaccine.** COVI-VAC is a "universal" booster, intranasal vaccine. Intranasal vaccines can address the primary needs of LMICs and may have a significant role to play in ending the pandemic (Waltz 2022).

   (a)   Dosage is 0.25 milliliters per nostril using nasal dropper.
   (b)   Dosage is two doses (28 days apart) for the primary series; one dose for the heterologous booster.
   (c)   Vaccine is refrigerator-stable for 1 month and/or residential freezer-stable for 3 years.

   Platform proof-of concept: Phase 1 demonstrated safety, genetic stability, broad immune response, and signal of efficacy:

   (a)   induced nAbs and conserved T-cell immunity (including Omicron); and
   (b)   demonstrated potential to block transmission of virus through nasal immunity.

**Partnered for development:** Codagenix has partnered with the Serum Institute of India Pvt. Ltd., which states it is the largest vaccine manufacturer in the world by doses sold and produced, as the manufacturer of COVI-VAC (CISION PR Newswire 2020).

**Phase 3 WHO Solidarity Trial Vaccines:** As of 2022, COVI-VAC was lined up for evaluation of primary efficacy supportive of National Regulatory Authority EUA and WHO EUL; Phase 1 heterologous booster study was underway.

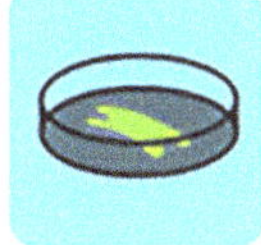

## 4. Vaccine Pipeline

Codagenix designs and develops several vaccine candidates in tandem, and uses rational, live virus vaccine technology considered to be globally scalable to address emerging public health threats (Table 7).

## Table 7: Vaccine Pipeline for Codagenix

| Vaccine Name | Indication Group | Development Stage | | | | | |
|---|---|---|---|---|---|---|---|
| | | Discovery | Preclinical | Phase 1 | Phase 2 | Phase 3 | Registration |
| CoviLiv | COVID-19 | ●━━━━━━━━━━━━━━━━━━● | | | | | |
| RSV CodaVax Adult | RSV | ●━━━━━━━━━━━● | | | | | |
| RSV CodaVax Pediatric | RSV | ●━━━━━● | | | | | |
| Universal influenza CodaVax-H1N1 | Influenza | ●━━━━━━━━━━━● | | | | | |
| Yellow Fever | Yellow Fever | ●━━━● | | | | | |
| CDX-DENV | Dengue Fever | ●━━━● | | | | | |
| CDX-ZKV | Zika Virus | ●━━━● | | | | | |

COVID-19 = coronavirus disease, RSV = respiratory syncytial virus.

Source: Codagenix.

(i)  **CodaVax-RSV: Live-Attenuated Vaccine for Prevention of Severe Respiratory Syncytial Virus Disease[2]**

   (a)  Genetically stable, live-attenuated vaccine among an array of single-antigen, antibody-focused developers (Le Nouën et al. 2017)

   (b)  Demonstrated safety in Phase 1 study of older people and signal of "must have" cell-mediated immunity (Cherukuri et al. 2013)

   (c)  Optionality for intranasal and injectable administration in infants, children, and older people where the burden of disease is highest
   - Preclinical animal models indicate robust antibody and T-cell responses

   (d)  Open US Food and Drug Administration (US FDA) Investigational New Drug with target Phase 1 clinical trial in pediatrics enrolling in 2023
   - 0.25 milliliters by nasal dropper per nostril
   - 1–2 dose regimens under evaluation

(ii)  **CodaVax-H1N1: Live-Attenuated Vaccine for Universal Influenza[3]**

   (a)  New live-attenuated mechanism-of-action and unique major antigen (HA) presentation may induce broadly nAbs, which increases cross-protection against mismatched strains (Impagliazzo et al. 2015)
   - Vast majority of licensed influenza vaccines are inactivated

   (b)  Optionality for intranasal and injectable administration in infants, children, adults, and older people
   - Preclinical animal models indicate robust antibody response exceeding WHO and US FDA established surrogate endpoint for licensure

   (c)  Ongoing Phase 1 injectable study in healthy adults

(iii)  **Yellow Fever: Live-Attenuated Vaccine for Dengue Fever[4]**

   (a)  Lead candidate, developed from WHO reference strain using Codagenix proprietary technology, attenuated and adapted for high-yield scale-up in modern animal-origin free Vero cell culture with genetic stability
   - Current Yellow Fever vaccines produced with decades-old chick embryo technology

---

[2]  See Mueller et al. (2020).
[3]  See Stauft et al. (2019).
[4]  See Stauft et al. (2018).

    (b)    WHO and US FDA established surrogate endpoint licensure (SEP)

    (c)    Demonstrated one-dose injectable preclinical immunogenicity achieving SEP in primates with viral attenuation superior to license product

**(iv)  CodaVax-DENV: Live-Attenuated Vaccine for Dengue Fever**

    (a)    Novel homologous tetravalent dengue serotypes 1, 2, 3, 4 and contemporary-to-current-circulating strains lead candidate developed
- Licensed and other under-development candidates are not wholly homologous to each serotype and are based on decades-old strains that may no longer be in circulation

    (b)    In vivo proof-of-concept for attenuation and balancing of immunogenicity in small animals and primates

    (c)    The manufacturing process uses an animal-free origin Vero cell culture process that should allow for technical transfer in accordance with GMP requirements

    (d)    In development with support from the US Department of Defense (Codagenix 2022a)

**(v)  ZIKA: Live-Attenuated Vaccine for Zika Fever**

    (a)    In vivo proof-of-concept for attenuation, immunogenicity, and efficacy in primates

    (b)    Non-neurotropic in human cell lines

# G.  HDT Bio (United States)

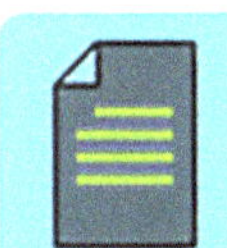

### 1. Background

HDT Bio is based in Seattle and began as an oncology startup in 2019, with infectious diseases becoming more of a recent company focus following the onset of the COVID-19 pandemic.

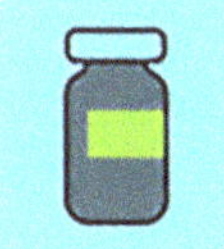

### 2. Vaccine Platform and Technologies

LION is the company's RNA delivery technology based on a proprietary lipid nanoparticle system tailored for rapid responses to emerging infectious diseases and personalized interventions for oncology patients (Erasmus et al. 2020). The LION platform allows disease antigens or immune stimulants to reach and be expressed by target cells through protecting and stabilizing replicating RNA. After expression, antigens and stimulants jointly magnify the immune response in a highly specific manner to help the body respond to existing diseases and may also offer immunity against future infection. The LION platform avoids costly or constrained ingredients to meet global demand.

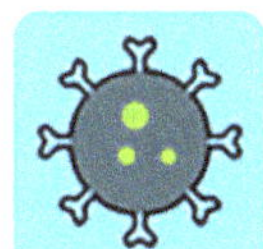

### 3. COVID-19 Vaccine

Also known as Gemcovac-19, HDT-301 is a self-amplifying RNA (saRNA) COVID-19 vaccine that has obtained EUA from the Indian regulator (Pharmaceutical Technology 2022). The saRNA vaccine technology replicates itself following administration and is thus effective at extremely low doses: up to 20 times lower than current vaccines. In addition, it is stable at ordinary refrigerator temperatures (between 2°C and 8°C).

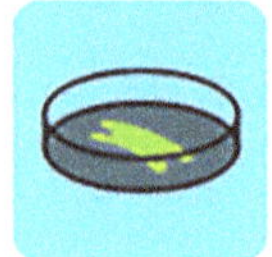

## 4. Vaccine Pipeline

Working with global partners including Gennova Biopharmaceuticals (India), SENAI CIMATEC (Brazil), and Quratis (Republic of Korea), HDT Bio has several vaccines in its developmental pipeline (Table 8).

### Table 8: Vaccine Pipeline for HDT Bio

| Vaccine Name | Indication Group | Development Stage | | | | | |
|---|---|---|---|---|---|---|---|
| | | Discovery | Preclinical | Phase 1 | Phase 2 | Phase 3 | Registration |
| HDT-301 | COVID-19 | ●————————————————————● | | | | | |
| HGCO19 | RSV | ●————————————————————————————————————————————————● |
| QTP5104 | RSV | ●————————————————————● | | | | | |
| RNA MCTI CIMATEC HDT | Influenza | ●————————————————————● | | | | | |
| HDT-311 | Yellow Fever | ●————————————● | | | | | |
| HDT-321 | Dengue Fever | ●——● | | | | | |
| HDT-331 | Zika Virus | ●——● | | | | | |

CCHFV = Crimean-Congo hemorrhagic fever, COVID-19 = coronavirus disease.

Source: HDT Bio.

(i)    **HDT-311.** Using the same antigen target as the market-leading shingles product Shingrix, this vaccine seeks to reduce costs and supply constraints. Preclinical data suggests that a single-shot administration may be sufficient to protect elderly patients from shingles.

(ii)    **HDT-321 and HDT-331.** These vaccines are under development to prevent neglected tropical diseases induced by zoonotic viruses that have been identified as potential emerging pandemic threats:

HDT-321 is for Crimean-Congo hemorrhagic fever virus (CCHFV). CCHFV is found and spread by ticks that feed on a variety of domestic and wild animals (Gholizadeh et al. 2022). People can be infected directly by ticks or through contact with products from infected animals. The disease can cause uncontrolled bleeding and has a high mortality (range: 9%–50%). The ticks can be found across Africa, central and southern Asia, and southeastern Europe.

HDT-331 is for Nipah virus (NiV). NiV is found in fruit bats that can spread the virus to pigs, people, and to date palm sap (Devnath et al. 2022). Annual outbreaks occur primarily in Bangladesh and India. Humans infected with NiV develop breathing difficulties and encephalitis with death occurring in around 40%–75%.

There are no approved vaccines for these viruses. However, the University of Texas Medical Branch was recently awarded funding from the US government to collaborate with HDT Bio to develop an saRNA vaccine platform technology for emerging viral threats. The funding supports the development of vaccines for CCHFV and NiV to the end of Phase 1 clinical trials.

(iii)    **HDT-201.** Although not a vaccine, this product uses constructed RNAs to activate a receptor on most cells in the body called the RIG-I receptor that helps the immune system recognize that the cell is infected by a virus (Esser-Nobis et al. 2020). Activation of the RIG-I signaling pathway triggers the immune system to destroy infected cells (Lee et al. 2021).

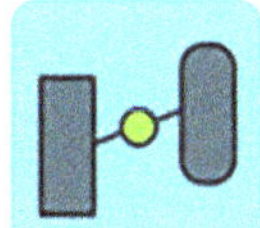

### 5. Partnerships and/or Approach to Working with Low- and Middle-Income Countries

In 2012, 65% of all deaths from cancer worldwide were in low- and middle-income countries (LMICs) (Parkin et al. 2005). This is expected to increase to 75% by 2030 (*The Lancet* 2018). Around 70% of cancer patients in LMICs are diagnosed at a late stage—in these cases, half of the patients do not even receive palliative care (Poudel et al. 2019). HDT Bio's technologies provide therapeutic options for oncology patients. Junction openers, immune activators, and cancer vaccines are tumor-agnostic and may be used broadly for a range of organs and tissues (Yumul et al. 2016; Pitner et al. 2019).

Infectious diseases and antimicrobial resistance are also significant future health-care concerns. Health care-associated infections account for high rates of morbidity and mortality worldwide, with LMICs disproportionately affected by adverse outcomes (Maki and Zervos 2021). The company's immune activators and RNA-based vaccines (Fuller and Berglund 2020) may be well suited to address unmet needs in LMICs in a cost-effective way, with vaccine pricing set according to the local economics in specific regions.

# H.  Medigen Vaccine Biologics Corp (Taipei,China)

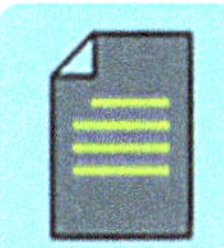

### 1. Background

Medigen Vaccine Biologics Corp (MVC) is a Taipei,China-based biopharmaceutical company founded in 2012, focused on the development and mass production of vaccines and biologics. MVC has GMP cell culture mass production facilities manufacturing vaccines licensed by the Food and Drug Administration of Taipei,China.

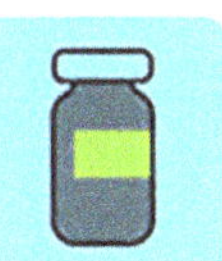

### 2. Vaccine Platforms and Technologies

MVC specializes in mammalian cell culture processes and operates Taipei,China's large-scale Pharmaceutical Inspection Co-operation Scheme (PIC/S) GMP cell culture manufacturing plant for the mass production of viral vaccines. This includes two separate production lines certified to Biosafety Level 2 for the production of vaccines and antibodies. MVC also has quality control and R&D labs.

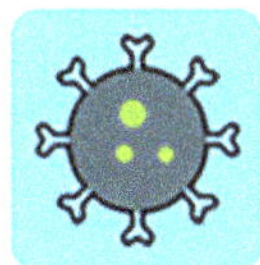

### 3. COVID-19 Vaccines

MVC COVID-19 vaccine is a Chinese hamster ovary cell-derived spike protein (subunit) vaccine that contains the recombinant spike protein (S-2P) of the SARS-CoV-2 virus (Kuo et al. 2020; Lien et al. 2021; Hsieh et al. 2021a, 2021b, 2022; C. E. Lien et al. 2022; Kuo et al. 2022a; Y. Lien et al. 2022; Waits et al. 2022; Lin et al. 2022; Estrada et al. 2022; Cheng et al. 2021). The S-2P antigen is licensed by the US National Institutes of Health. The vaccine also uses adjuvants of aluminum hydroxide and CpG 1018 (developed by Dynavax). The dosage schedule is two doses, 28 days apart, and is currently indicated for individuals 20 years of age and above. The vaccine is administered intramuscularly and can be stored between 2°C and 8°C for 1 year and is available as a prefilled syringe or in multidose vials. Further studies are planned and ongoing to obtain pediatric and adolescent authorization.

MVC COVID-19 vaccine was granted an EUA by the Food and Drug Administration of Taipei,China in July 2021. Since then, it was granted EUA in Eswatini, Paraguay, and Somaliland. Currently, regulatory applications are underway for the US FDA, European Medicines Agency, Therapeutic Goods Administration (TGA) in Australia, and WHO EUL. The vaccine was selected as one of WHO's Solidarity Trial Vaccines in 2021 (BioPharmaAPAC 2021). The vaccine was one of four vaccines rolled out as part of Taipei,China's initial vaccination program in 2021 (Chuang et al. 2022) along with Comirnaty/BNT162b2 (Pfizer-BioNTech), Spikevax/mRNA-1273 (Moderna), and Vaxzevria/ChAdOx1 (AstraZeneca).

The company has recently published preclinical data on its bivalent vaccine against Omicron subvariants (Kuo et al. 2022b).

A review by the Food and Drug Administration of Taipei,China found that three doses of the MVC COVID-19 vaccine provided over 90% efficacy against death and severe illness. The analysis using data collected from March 2021 to September 2022 compared the effectiveness of three MVC COVID-19 vaccine doses with three doses of three other COVID-19 vaccines for all age groups:

(i)   For efficacy in preventing death from COVID-19:

    (a)   Medigen (MVC COVID-19) = 90.3%
    (b)   Pfizer-BioNTech (Comirnaty/BNT162b2) = 95.6%
    (c)   Moderna (Spikevax/mRNA-1273) = 90%
    (d)   AstraZeneca (Vaxzevria/ChAdOx1) = 60.9%

(ii)  For efficacy in avoiding moderate to severe disease from COVID-19 infection:

    (a)   Medigen (MVC COVID-19) = 91.4%
    (b)   Pfizer-BioNTech (Comirnaty/BNT162b2) = 95.8%
    (c)   Moderna (Spikevax/mRNA-1273) = 87.4%
    (d)   AstraZeneca (Vaxzevria/ChAdOx1) = 65.9%

The reports were verified using 2 years' data from the national systems for vaccination and disease notifications for 23 million people.

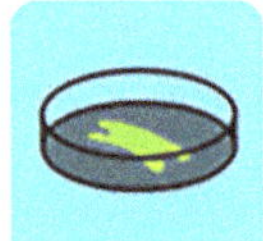

## 4.  Vaccine Pipeline

MVC has numerous vaccines in various stages of clinical trial or regulatory approval, which include vaccines against influenza, dengue fever, Japanese encephalitis, and tuberculosis. The company's two most advanced vaccines are against COVID-19 and enterovirus A71 (Table 9).

Envacgen is an enterovirus A71 vaccine with clinical data for infants aged 2–6 months (Huang et al. 2019; T. T. Nguyen et al. 2022). Envacgen is also an effective preventive agent in controlling enterovirus infection with severe complications. Enterovirus A71 is significantly more pathogenic than other known enteroviruses, especially for neurological complications (Li et al. 2021). Children under the age of 5 years are especially prone to critical complications and death.

Envacgen is an inactivated whole virus vaccine with an efficacy against enterovirus A71 infection of at least 96.8%. Delivered by intramuscular injection, two doses are required, 56 days apart. For infants who received the first dose under 2 years of age, a third booster dose should be given after 1 year from the first shot to retain the best protection.

Table 9: Vaccine Pipeline for Medigen Vaccine Biologics Corp.

| Vaccine Name | Indication Group | Discovery | Preclinical | Phase 1 | Phase 2 | Phase 3 | Registration |
|---|---|---|---|---|---|---|---|
| Inactivated EV-A71 | Enterovirus | | | | | | |
| CA16 + EV-A71 VLP | Influenza | | | | | | |
| Inactivated H5N1 | Influenza | | | | | | |
| Inactivated H7N9 | Influenza | | | | | | |
| Inactivated QIV | Influenza | N/A | | | | | |
| Tetravalent Attenuated Vaccine | Dengue Fever | | | | | | |
| Inactivated whole virus | Japanese Encephalitis | | | | | | |
| Palivizumab mAb | N/A | | | | | | |
| BCG | Tuberculosis | N/A | | | | | |
| Snake anti-venom | Venom | N/A | | | | | |
| Spike Protein (S-2P) | COVID-19 | | | | | | |

COVID-19 = coronavirus disease, N/A = not applicable.

Source: Medigen Vaccine Biologics Corp.

## 5. Partnerships and/or Approach to Working with Low- and Middle-Income Countries

MVC is offering technology access to its products and turnkey solutions for cell-based vaccine manufacturing, combining its factory design with the accompanying PIC/S GMP documentation package for LMICs. The company has made contractual commitments to WHO and the Coalition for Epidemic Preparedness Innovations to make both the MVC COVID-19 and Envacgen vaccines accessible and affordable to LMICs. MVC joined a consortium of LMICs in 2016 to develop palivizumab against the respiratory syncytial virus. According to Li et al. (2022), LMICs have the overwhelming burden of disease attributable to RSV, including almost all reported lower respiratory infections (95%) and deaths (97%).

# I. Nanogen Pharmaceutical Biotechnology (Viet Nam)

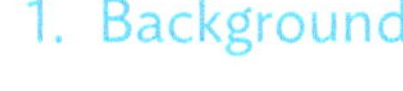

## 1. Background

Based in Viet Nam and established in 1997, Nanogen Pharmaceutical Biotechnology develops therapeutic products based on advanced recombinant DNA or protein technology. Nanogen's drug discovery focuses on the development of recombinant antibodies, cytokines, hormones, chemotherapy medications, and vaccines. Nanogen has developed gene-to-therapy biopharmaceuticals for the treatment of anemia, cancers, and Hepatitis B and C. Nanogen has also been conducting clinical trials on monoclonal antibodies for oncology immunotherapy and COVID-19 vaccines and treatments.

Nanogen's facilities include four factories and one R&D center located across three provinces of Viet Nam. The company states it has a manufacturing capacity of more than 100 million products yearly, and that it has already supplied products to countries across Africa, Asia, Europe, and North America.

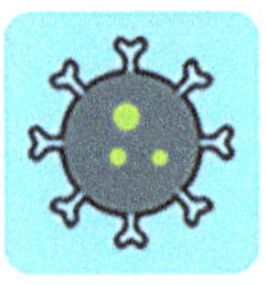

### 2. COVID-19 Vaccine

Nanocovax is Nanogen's protein subunit COVID-19 vaccine developed in 2020; this was following an approach by the Ministry of Health for a domestically produced vaccine. A subunit vaccine contains harmless antigen fragments (proteins) of the SARS-CoV-2 virus that induce a protective immune response. In Nanocovax, the transmembrane domain of the S protein was removed, with the S protein produced using recombinant DNA or protein technology on Chinese hamster ovary cells (Tran et al. 2021; T. P. Nguyen et al. 2022a). To boost immune response, an aluminum adjuvant is used in the Nanocovax vaccine.

A Phase 3 clinical trial run in Viet Nam during the 2021 Delta wave showed that Nanocovax had a 51.5% efficacy against symptomatic COVID-19 and 93.3% against hospitalization and/or death (T.P. Nguyen et al. 2022b). Adverse events were uncommon, minor (fatigue and muscle aches), and similar to rates observed in those who received the placebo. Another Phase 3 clinical trial finalized in 2022 showed that Nanocovax (25 micrograms, regimen of two injections 28 days apart) met all safety criteria. The immunogenicity was high when compared with the placebo: 99.2% of subjects had seroconverted (a fourfold increase over placebo), with the proportion of study subjects having high virus neutralizing activity (98.8%) at 42 days after injection. The rate of seroconversion in the vaccine group at 6 months remained high (94.7%). The protective efficacy of Nanocovax against COVID-19 with severe clinical symptoms and death was 96%, which is comparable with already-approved vaccines: Comirnaty/ BNT162b2 (Pfizer-BioNTech) of 95%, Spikevax/mRNA-1273 (Moderna) of 98%, and Vaxzevria/ChAdOx1 (AstraZeneca) of 90% (Nasreen et al. 2022). The protective efficacy of Nanocovax against clinically symptomatic COVID-19 of any severity gradually decreased over time: from 90% at 2 months to 47% at 5 months. In summary, Nanocovax met the protocol's criteria for safety, immunogenicity, and protective efficacy.

The storage of Nanocovax between 2°C and 8°C is also compatible with ordinary refrigeration. The company states that currently, its bioreactors have a manufacturing capacity of 10–20 million Nanocovax doses monthly, which satisfies domestic demand and allows for export. Nanocovax costs around $5.00 per dose (Bastian 2022).

# J.  Providence Therapeutics (Canada)

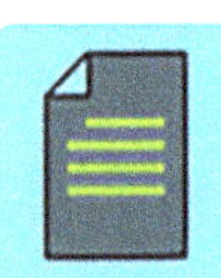

### 1. Background

Providence Therapeutics is a Canadian biotechnology company founded in 2015 that specializes in messenger RNA (mRNA) vaccine therapies.

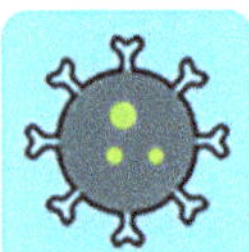

### 2. COVID-19 Vaccine

In partnership with Genevant, a company specializing in lipid nanoparticle (LNP) technology, Providence developed PTX-COVID19-B as an LNP-formulated, nucleoside-modified mRNA vaccine encoding for D614G SARS-CoV-2 spike glycoprotein. It is stable at minus 20°C for 12 months.

Phase 1 clinical trials of the PTX-COVID19-B vaccine against COVID-19 were initiated in January 2021, with the vaccine accepted into the WHO Solidarity Trial Vaccines in December 2021. Phase 1 results showed no serious adverse events. Minor events were mostly related to local issues at the site of vaccine administration and other mild reactions such as fever and fatigue. There were high titers of anti-receptor binding domain (RBD), anti-S protein IgG, and neutralization titers, along with 100% seroconversion after the first immunization. The results showed strong neutralization titers against the original Wuhan strain and some variants of concern (Alpha,

Beta, Delta), including T-cell response. High levels of antibodies were detected 20 weeks after the second immunization with persistent anti-S and anti-RBD responses (Liu et al. 2022; Orozco et al. 2022).

Phase 2 comparator clinical trials, comparing PTX-COVID19-B to the Comirnaty (Pfizer-BioNTech) mRNA vaccine, were finalized in 2022. The Providence Therapeutic vaccine was noninferior for the geometric mean titer ratio of nAbs observed. PTX-COVID19-B was also similar to Comirnaty in terms of safety and tolerability.

During 2023, Providence will initiate heterologous Phase 3 comparator booster trials of PTX-COVID19-B versus Comirnaty (Pfizer-BioNTech) or Vaxzevria (AstraZeneca), followed by booster indication with PTX-COVID19-M1, a bivalent vaccine that combines two mRNAs (PTX-COVID19-B and Omicron variant). Commercial production of PTX-COVID19-B is scheduled for 2023.

A third mRNA vaccine formulation, PTX-COVID19-LT, takes different parts of the SARS-CoV-2 virus that are better conserved than the S glycoprotein to generate a stronger T-cell response and establish better long-term immunity.

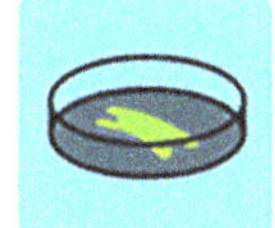

## 3.  Vaccine Pipeline

Providence has a vaccine pipeline designed against infectious diseases such as COVID-19 and influenza, as well as oncology vaccines (Table 10).

### Table 10: Vaccine Pipeline for Providence Therapeutics

| Vaccine Name | Indication Group | Development Stage | | | | | |
|---|---|---|---|---|---|---|---|
| | | Discovery | Preclinical | Phase 1 | Phase 2 | Phase 3 | Registration |
| PTX-COVID19-B | COVID-19 | | | | ● | | |
| PTX-COVID19-B Booster | COVID-19 | | | | | ● | |
| PTX-COVID19-M1 Omicron bivalent | COVID-19 | ● | | | | | |
| PTX-COVID19-LT Multivalent | COVID-19 | ● | | | | | |
| EP-A | N/A | ● | | | | | |
| EP-B | N/A | ● | | | | | |
| PTX-FLU | Influenza | ● | | | | | |
| PTX-C | N/A | ● | | | | | |
| PTX-102 | Cancer | ● | | | | | |
| PTX-103 | Cancer | ● | | | | | |
| PTX-104 | Cancer | ● | | | | | |
| PTX-105 | Cancer | ● | | | | | |

COVID-19 = coronavirus disease, N/A = not applicable.

Source: Medigen Vaccine Biologics Corp.

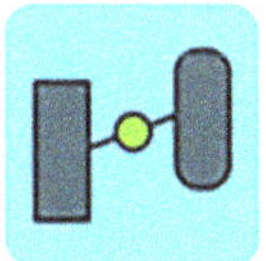

## 4.  Partnerships and/or Approach to Working with Low- and Middle-Income Countries

The company's mission is to develop an mRNA platform that enables developers through collaborations and partnerships to produce affordably priced vaccines, including for low- and middle-income countries.

In 2021, Providence entered a commercial alliance with a company from the PRC, Everest Medicines. This alliance consists of two components:

(i)    regional licensing of mRNA COVID-19 vaccine candidates in developing markets in Asia, including Pakistan, the PRC, and Southeast Asia; and

(ii)   licensing the mRNA technology platform to other products.

The mRNA formulation and process scale-up capability to the kilogram scale has been developed and is being transferred to contract development and manufacturing companies. Manufacturing technology transfer to these companies has been accomplished with additional technology transfers now underway to Everest. Everest is opening a manufacturing facility in Jiashan, Zhejiang Province, with a declared capacity of 500–600 million doses annually. Characterization of the vaccine product illustrates comparability of all scales produced to date (Table 11):

#### Table 11: Scale up of mRNA Vaccine Manufacturing Capacity for Providence Therapeutics

| Scale | Drug Substance | Drug Product | Fill-finish |
|---|---|---|---|
| Clinical scale | 100 ml/500 mg IVT reaction (~70% yield) | 300 mg formulation (50%–70% yield) | 500 vials 5,000 doses |
| Mid-scale | 1.25 l / 5 g IVT reaction (~75% yield) | 4 g formulation (75%–80% yield) | 7,000 vials 70,000 doses |
| Commercial scale | 25 l / 125 g IVT (~80% yield) | 4 x 30 g formulation (~80% yield) | 60 g yields 1,000,000 doses |

g = grams, IVT = in vitro transcription, l = liter, mg = milligrams, ml = milliliters.
Source: Providence Therapeutics.

# K.  Raphael Labs (Ireland)

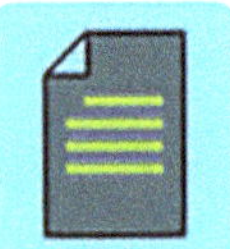

## 1. Background

With a view to using prophylaxis as a key strategy in controlling the future spread of airborne respiratory viruses, Raphael Labs has developed nasal sprays to work against multiple virus strains and complement traditional vaccines and personal protective equipment. The Ireland-based company was founded in 2020.

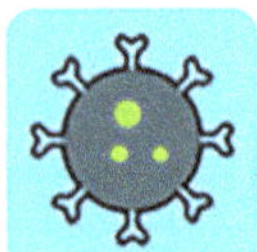

## 2. COVID-19 Vaccine

Coronaviruses and influenza viral infections usually start in the nasal epithelia via cellular processes that prime binding and entry of viruses to host cells. Optimizing the local environment in the nasal cavity through a nasal spray may maintain homeostasis and prevent viruses from replicating in cells (Fuentes-Prior et al. 2021).

pHOXWELL is a prophylactic nasal spray that combines natural virucides with a novel scientific platform. Its base solution is Vita Raphael, which mimics the body's interstitial fluid and is claimed to offer up to 8 hours of protection from SARS-CoV-2 viral infection per application. In a real-world trial in India, during the 2021 Delta outbreak (Balmforth et al. 2022), health-care workers who had not been infected with or vaccinated against

COVID-19 were randomized to use either the pHOXWELL nasal spray or a placebo three times each day for 45 days. There were no serious adverse effects and a difference in the proportion of health-care workers who had been infected (measured by COVID-19 antibodies) was observed—13.1% in those who used the pHOXWELL spray versus 34.5% who took the placebo. The company reports that this corresponds to the pHOXWELL nasal spray reducing the number of SARS-CoV-2 infections by 62%. In addition, Raphael Labs believes that pHOXWELL's mode of action may also block transmission of the SARS-CoV-2 virus between individuals.

pHOXWELL is engineered to complement personal protective equipment use and vaccination. It is also aimed at those who are yet to be vaccinated or cannot be vaccinated (Table 12).

### Table 12: Gaps in Measures to Prevent Respiratory Infections

| Standard Care | Major Gaps |
|---|---|
| Prophylaxis medicines | • None identified for coronaviruses and rhinoviruses<br>• Routine influenza prophylaxis not recommended |
| Vaccines to prevent disease | • None for rhinoviruses, coronaviruses, (except SARS-CoV-2)<br>• Modest efficacy against influenza<br>• Supply challenges in warm climates, rural areas<br>• Poor access in developing countries<br>• Hesitancy to use<br>• Do not prevent viral infiltration<br>• Insufficient alone |
| Use of personal protective equipment to prevent transmission | • Insufficiently effective<br>• Failure to use, incorrect use, and malfunction<br>• Poor availability in many settings and countries<br>• Inadequate alone |
| Good hygiene | • Poor understanding of good measures<br>• Inconvenient access to hygiene aids<br>• Unreliable |
| Social distancing and isolation | • Impractical in many situations<br>• Low acceptance, especially over time<br>• Not suitable over the long term<br>• Unsustainable |

SARS-CoV-2 = severe acute respiratory syndrome coronavirus 2.
Source: Raphael Labs.

Approximately one in 8 people infected with the SARS-CoV-2 virus progresses to develop long COVID-19 (Ballering et al. 2022), with persistent symptoms for 3 months or more. Those with preexisting medical conditions are more likely to develop the condition (Yoo et al. 2022), with the most common symptoms being fatigue and memory problems (C. Chen et al. 2022). Since the pHOXWELL prophylactic spray reduces the incidence of SARS-CoV-2 infections, the company states that it may also prevent associated health conditions expressed through long COVID-19.

pHOXWELL is stable at room temperature and requires no refrigeration throughout the supply chain. Simple manufacturing and distribution enable rapid emergency deployment for current and future virus outbreaks in countries of need.

Raphael Labs is applying for market authorization via the Provisional Registration Pathway (accelerated review) by the Therapeutic Goods Administration (Australia). The United Kingdom (UK) regulator, the Medicines and Healthcare Products Regulatory Agency (MHRA) said that pHOXWELL was ready for Phase 3 clinical trials and that one of the innovative regulatory pathways for faster assessment would be appropriate.

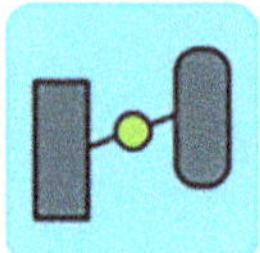

### 3. Partnerships and/or Approach to Working with Low- and Middle-Income Countries

The company believes that LMICs in Asia could benefit from the use of a simple prophylactic nasal spray against the SARS-CoV-2 virus due to the region's large populations, low overall vaccination rates, and more vulnerable health-care systems.

# L.  Sanofi (France)

### 1. Background

Sanofi is a French multinational pharmaceutical and health-care company with multiple good manufacturing practice (GMP) manufacturing sites. Sanofi says it supplies over 2.5 million doses of vaccines every day. The company offers a range of vaccines for the following infectious diseases:

(i)     Diphtheria, Haemophilus influenzae type b (Hib), Hepatitis A, Hepatitis B, Pertussis, Poliomyelitis, Tetanus,
(ii)    Meningococcal, Meningitis
(iii)   Yellow fever, Rabies, Japanese encephalitis, typhoid fever, dengue
(iv)    Influenza (Flublok Quadrivalent)[5]
(v)     Respiratory syncytial virus (RSV)
(vi)    COVID-19

Research and development priorities include the following:

(i)     New vaccine candidates: RSV vaccines for toddlers and older adults, next generation influenza vaccines
(ii)    Investing in mRNA to deliver innovative next generation vaccines, starting with influenza
(iii)   Opening new growth areas: chlamydia (de la Maza, Darville, and Pal 2021) and acne vaccines
(iv)    Expanding the company's approach with established platforms
(v)     Innovation in vaccines manufacturing

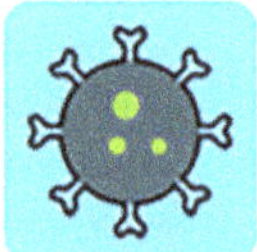

### 2. COVID-19 Vaccine

Sanofi has successfully developed a second-generation COVID-19 vaccine, VidPrevtyn Beta, which is based on the SARS-CoV-2 Beta variant antigen. The vaccine was developed using a licensed recombinant vaccine platform (also used for Flublok) and requires normal refrigeration (between 2°C and 8°C).

---

5    Government of Australia, Department of Health and Aged Care. Flublok Quadrivalent. https://www.tga.gov.au/resources/auspmd/flublok-quadrivalent.

Vidprevtyn Beta is a monovalent, recombinant, protein-based vaccine with a synthetic version of the spike (S) protein found on the surface of the SARS-CoV-2 virus. The S protein stimulates the immune system to produce nAbs that protect the body from COVID-19 infection. The vaccine is formulated, in combination with an adjuvant, to help strengthen the immune responses to the vaccine (Francica et al. 2021; Goepfert et al. 2021; Sridhar et al. 2022; Pavot et al. 2022).

The vaccine was approved by the European Medicines Agency in 2022 as a booster dose for adults (18 years and over) in those who have already been given either an adenoviral or mRNA COVID-19 vaccine (European Medicines Agency 2022a).

The vaccine led to a strong and broad immune response in registration studies (two immunogenicity studies and a Phase 3 primary efficacy trial) conducted when Omicron strains were dominant. Used as a booster dose after a primary course (two doses) of Comirnaty, VidPrevtyn Beta generated higher levels of nAb than booster doses of either Comirnaty or the first-generation of the Sanofi-GSK vaccine. Both vaccines were developed for the original COVID-19 strain (called D164).

For adults aged between 18 and 73 years, nAbs against Omicron BA.1 and BA.4/BA.5 were about 2.5 times higher for VidPrevtyn Beta than when Comirnaty was used as the booster dose.

For adults aged 18-55 years, a booster dose of VidPrevtyn Beta increased antibody titers by a factor of 13 for the original D614 strain and by 34 for the Beta strain. Adverse reactions were generally mild to moderate and self-limiting.

The efficacy of VidPrevtyn Beta in preventing COVID-19 infection, following a primary course of a bivalent (D164 and Beta strains) COVID-19 vaccine, was examined in a randomized, double-blind, placebo-controlled trial. The trial found that the vaccine had a 64.7% efficacy against symptomatic infection in adults irrespective of whether they had ever been infected with COVID-19, whereas efficacy was 75.1% in people who had been infected before vaccination.

# M.  Shionogi (Japan)

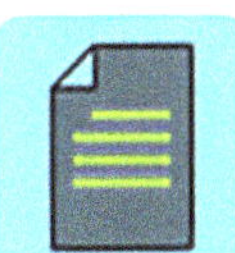

### 1.  Background

Shionogi is a global pharmaceutical company founded in 1878 with headquarters in Osaka, Japan. Shionogi has developed pharmaceutical products to treat Alzheimer's disease, attention deficit hyperactivity disorder, chronic liver disease, and infectious diseases.

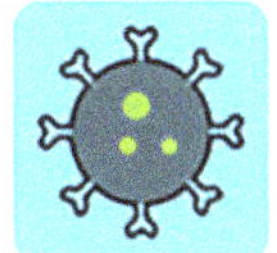

### 2.  COVID-19 Vaccine

The S-268019 recombinant protein vaccine comprises a modified recombinant spike protein (S-2P) of the SARS-CoV-2 virus made via a baculovirus expression system in insect cells and combined with a squalene-based adjuvant (Iwata et al. 2022; Hashimoto et al. 2022; Shinkai et al. 2022). The S-268019 vaccine is in Phase 3 clinical trials in Japan and Viet Nam. The vaccine, administered intramuscularly, can be stored using ordinary refrigeration temperatures (2°C to 8°C), which avoids freezing and thawing. In November 2022, Shionogi filed for regulatory approval with Japan's Pharmaceuticals and Medical Devices Agency (Shionogi 2022).

Shionogi is expanding its facilities and improving its methods to enable large-scale manufacturing. Shionogi is also partnering with Api Co Ltd. and UNIGEN Inc. to develop and sustain a manufacturing capacity of over 60 million doses yearly.

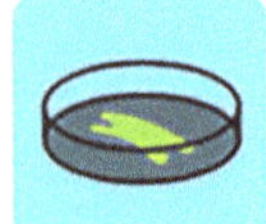

### 3. Vaccine Pipeline

In Japan, Shionogi is collaborating with Chiba University Hospital and HanaVax Inc. to develop a nasal COVID-19 vaccine using a cationic nanogel delivery system. Nasal vaccines may prevent infection and interrupt further transmission by enhancing immunity in the upper airways. They avoid injection, could be administered by health staff with lower levels of training, and delivered even in basic health systems. This makes nasal vaccines ideal for low- and middle-income countries.

# N.  Valneva (France)

### 1. Background

Valneva is a French company focused on vaccines for infectious diseases. Valneva has successfully commercialized three vaccines, including for COVID-19, and rapidly advanced a broad range of vaccine candidates into clinical trials against Lyme disease and the Chikungunya virus, among other infectious diseases. In addition to France, Valneva is also present in Austria, Canada, Sweden, the UK, and the US.

Viral vaccines are manufactured in Valneva's facility in Livingston, Scotland, which is dedicated to drug substance production for the company's viral vaccines and has been producing travel vaccines for more than a decade. Vaccines produced by Valneva are approved by worldwide regulators, including the European Medicines Agency (EMA), MHRA, and the US FDA. The company has a second manufacturing site in Solna, Sweden, and dedicated GMP facilities in Vienna, Austria.

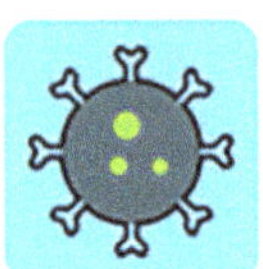

### 2. COVID-19 Vaccine

VLA2001 is an inactivated whole virus COVID-19 vaccine that contains virus with a high density of S proteins. Because it uses the entire COVID-19 virus and not just a component (such as vaccines targeting the S protein), VLA2001 potentially boosts T-cell responses against multiple structural proteins of the virus. The vaccine incorporates two adjuvants—Alum and CpG 1018—that have been repeatedly shown in preclinical studies to be superior to Alum alone in terms of antibody levels produced and the duration of T-cell responses.

VLA2001 is the first inactivated whole virus COVID-19 vaccine approved in Europe for a primary course (two doses given 28 days or more apart) in people aged between 18 and 50 years. In 2022, VLA2001 received standard marketing authorization in Europe through the EMA (European Medicines Agency 2022b) and conditional marketing authorization in the UK through the MHRA (Mahase et al. 2022). VLA2001 also received EUA in Bahrain and the United Arab Emirates. WHO has recommended the use of VLA2001 as either a primary vaccine or booster dose (Munro et al. 2021).

These regulatory approvals have come following numerous extensive clinical trials (Lazarus et al. 2022b). Pivotal Phase 3 clinical trials showed superiority of VLA2001 versus Vaxzevria (AstraZeneca), along with a more favorable tolerability (Lazarus et al. 2022a). VLA2001 has been shown to neutralize Delta and Omicron variants of concern in laboratory studies. The company has reported positive homologous and heterologous booster data.

The storage temperature for VLA2001 is standard refrigeration (between 2°C and 8°C). The shelf life is currently 15 months but is anticipated to be 24 months or longer.

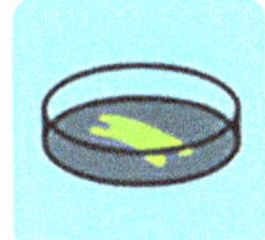

## 3. Vaccine Pipeline

Valneva has vaccines for Japanese encephalitis, cholera, and COVID-19 that have been authorized for use in various jurisdictions. Valneva also has several other products in advanced stages of development (Table 13).

### Table 13: Vaccine Pipeline for Valneva

| Vaccine Name | Indication Group | Development Stage | | | | | |
|---|---|---|---|---|---|---|---|
| | | Discovery | Preclinical | Phase 1 | Phase 2 | Phase 3 | Registration |
| VLA1553[2] | Chikungunya Virus | ━ | ━ | ━ | ━ | ● | |
| VLA15[3] | Lyme Disease | ━ | ━ | ━ | ━ | ● | |
| VLA84 | C. diff | ━ | ━ | ━ | ● | | |
| VLA1601 | Zika Virus | ━ | ━ | ━ | ● | | |
| VLA1554 | hMPV | ━ | ● | | | | |
| VLA2112 | Epstein-Barr Virus | ━ | ● | | | | |
| IXIARO | Japanese Encephalitis | ━ | ━ | ━ | ━ | ━ | ● |
| DUKORAL | Cholera + ETEC | ━ | ━ | ━ | ━ | ━ | ● |
| VLA2201 | COVID-19 | ━ | ━ | ━ | ━ | ━ | ● |

COVID-19 = coronavirus disease, ETEC = Enterotoxigenic Escherichia coli, hMPV = Human metapneumovirus.

Source: Valneva.

(i) **Ixiaro: Japanese encephalitis vaccine.** Approved for use in numerous territories including in Europe by the EMA (European Medicines Agency 2022c) and by the US FDA,[6] Ixiaro is used for people aged 2 months and older to protect against Japanese encephalitis. This virus is spread by mosquitoes that are found in rural areas throughout Asia. It can cause inflammation of the brain (encephalitis) and is fatal in about 25% of cases (Cramer et al. 2016; Taucher, Kollaritsch, and Dubischar 2019; Dubischar et al. 2017a, 2017b; Kadlecek et al. 2018; Jelinek et al. 2018; Schlegl et al. 2015; Eder et al. 2011; Dubischar-Kastner et al. 2010a, 2010b; Kaltenbock et al. 2009, 2010; Schuller et al. 2008a, 2008b, 2009, 2011; Tauber et al. 2007, 2008; Kollaritsch, Paulke-Korinek, and Dubischar-Kastner 2009). Ixiaro triggers the production of antibodies against the Japanese encephalitis virus and is given by intramuscular injection.

(ii) **Dukoral: Cholera vaccine.** Approved for use in numerous territories including in Europe by the EMA (Lazarus et al. 2022a and by the UK MHRA,[7] Dukoral is an oral vaccine used in people 2 years and older who are at risk of being infected with cholera. Cholera is bacterial infection from contaminated water or food that can cause life-threatening diarrhea (Shaikh et al. 2020; Pastor, Pedraz and Esquisabel 2013). Dukoral is an inactivated vaccine combined with a fragment of the cholera toxin (B subunit) that stimulates antibodies that prevent the pathogen and the toxin from attaching to the intestinal wall and causing diarrhea.

---

Valneva has several vaccines currently in preclinical and clinical trials. The two most advanced vaccines are in Phase 3 clinical trials:

(i)    **VLA1553: Chikungunya Vaccine**[8]

   (a)    This Chikungunya virus is spread by the Aedes mosquito, which is found in tropical areas throughout the world. The disease is especially prevalent in Asia, Africa, and Latin America (Silva and Dermody 2017). Currently, there are no treatments or vaccines for this infection.
   (b)    VLA1553 is a live attenuated vaccine that aims to stimulate lasting immunity with a single injection. The US FDA and EMA have recognized the unmet need for a Chikungunya virus vaccine and put VLA1553 on an expedited pathway for development (Fast Track[9] in the US and PRIME[10] scheme in Europe).
   (c)    VLA1553 immunogenicity data reported a seroresponse rate in 98.9% of people following a single dose. All participants seroconverted 14 days after vaccination and immunity was sustained over time (seroconversion sustained at 12 months and a seroresponse rate of 96.3% of participants on Day 1,801).
   (d)    VLA1553 safety data reported that it is generally well tolerated with mild adverse events (headache, fatigue, and myalgia) reported in about half the people in the study.

(ii)    **VLA15: Lyme Disease**[11]

   (a)    VLA15 contains six serotypes of *Borrelia burgdorferi* bacteria and targets the outer surface protein A to help protect against Lyme disease. This disease is spread by ticks and causes fevers, muscle aches, fatigue, and a rash (erythema migrans) early in the illness. Untreated, the infection can cause arthritis, inflammation of the heart, brain, and spinal cord.
   (b)    Received Fast Track designation from the US FDA.
   (c)    No available treatment to protect against Lyme disease.
   (d)    VLA15 induces a strong immune response in adults aged between 18 and 65 years and in children aged between 5 and 17 years. For children, the vaccine produced a better immunogenicity profile in those who received two or three doses.
   (e)    VLA15 safety data reported that it is generally safe and well tolerated in all ages, with no serious adverse events.
   (f)    Valneva has an exclusive, worldwide partnership with Pfizer to develop VLA15.

## 4. Partnerships and/or Approach to Working with Low- and Middle-Income Countries

Using its vaccine technology, Valneva can offer technology transfer to LMICs with the potential to produce their own vaccines against COVID-19; seasonal influenza; Japanese encephalitis; Zika, a mosquito-borne disease associated with birth defects (Wressnigg et al. 2022); *Clostridium difficile*, which is a bacterium that leads to diarrhea and can cause sepsis and inflammation, perforation or abnormal dilation of the colon (Bezay et al. 2016); and other infectious diseases.

---

# O. Vaxxas (Australia)

### 1. Background

Vaxxas is an Australian biotechnology company focused on enhancing the performance of vaccines and increasing access to vaccination using needle-free high-density microarray patch (HD-MAP) technology (Forster and Junger 2022). Vaxxas states that its patch technology is a "platform technology" that can potentially deliver any vaccine to the human body.

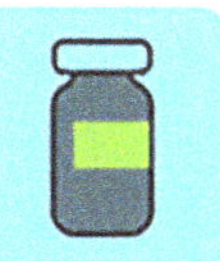

### 2. Vaccine Platforms and Technologies

**Vaccine patch technology.** HD-MAPs are small (1x1 centimeter) patches containing thousands of micro-projections (Forster et al. 2020). The vaccine is coated on the micro-projections and applied to the skin for a short period (around 10 seconds) using an applicator device made of aluminum and stainless steel. This design distributes the vaccine into the superficial layers of the skin that have high populations of antigen-presenting immune cells (Muller et al. 2020). The Vaxxas technology may offer advantages including dose sparing (Prow et al. 2010; Forster et al. 2020); thermostability (Pearson et al. 2013), which mitigates the need for cold-chain storage and distribution; reduced patient anxiety associated with traditional vaccination methods (Davies et al. 2022); low-skilled or self-administration; and lower cost per dose than traditional needle and syringe (Arya et al. 2016).

The company has published datasets, including preclinical and clinical studies, on the use of HD-MAP for vaccines for measles and rubella (Wan et al. 2021), influenza (Forster et al. 2020), and COVID-19 (McMillan et al. 2021). Results for an influenza vaccine showed that 1/6th of the standard dose used by the traditional needle and syringe delivery could induce a comparable immune response when delivered by HD-MAP.

Vaxxas manufactures the Hexapro SARS-CoV-2 spike vaccine patch in Phase 1 clinical trials. Studies testing COVID-19 vaccines using the HD-MAP technology on mice via the Hexapro SARS-CoV-2 spike vaccine patch showed enhanced immune response compared to needle and syringe, as well as being effective in combating COVID-19 variants of concern.

# P. Vaxxinity (United States)

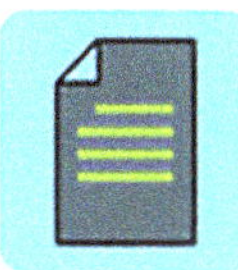

### 1. Background

Vaxxinity is a US biotechnology company that is developing synthetic peptide vaccines for infectious diseases like COVID-19, as well as chronic diseases, including Alzheimer's disease, hypercholesterolemia, migraines, and Parkinson's disease.

Chronic diseases are now responsible for more human deaths than infectious diseases (Stuckler et al. 2008). In 2019, seven out of the 10 leading causes of death were noncommunicable diseases, with lower respiratory infections ranked as the deadliest communicable disease in the world (WHO 2020). One reason for this shift is that vaccines have been so successful in preventing infectious diseases. WHO reports that licensed vaccines are available to prevent or contribute to the prevention and control, of 31 vaccine-preventable infections (WHO 2012).

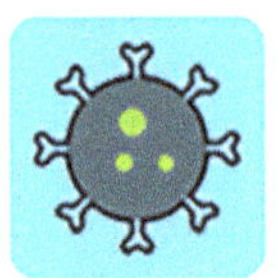

## 2. COVID-19 Vaccine

Vaxxinity's UB-612 vaccine has been designed and tested for booster immunization to mRNA, adeno-vectored, and inactivated COVID-19 vaccines.

Currently, UB-612 is being tested in Phase 3 multicountry clinical trial in over 1,000 subjects to evaluate the ability to boost immune responses stimulated by previous immunization with globally authorized COVID-19 vaccines manufactured using mRNA, adenovirus, or inactivated virus platforms. The vaccine is administered intramuscularly and has a shelf life of at least 24 months at ordinary refrigeration temperatures (2°C to 8°C), which avoids freezing and thawing.

The UB-612 vaccine contains a combination of subunit protein and synthetic peptide antigens. The UB-612 subunit protein—the receptor binding domain (RBD)—is essential for virus attachment to human cells, with most protective SARS-CoV-2 antibodies directed against the RBD. UB-612 also contains synthetic peptides, including epitopes from nucleocapsid, spike, and membrane, to activate durable B- and T-cell immunity to SARS-CoV-2. Before application to UB-612, the peptide vaccine technology was scientifically validated and successfully applied in veterinary health, with over 6 billion doses commercialized (Parrish 2022). Through the use of established technological platforms and ordinary refrigeration, UB-612 may be more affordable to LMICs to both purchase and store.

Animal trials showed that UB-612 led to high levels of nAbs and T-cell responses. This reduced viral loads, improved lung pathology scores, and slowed the disease progression after the animals were exposed to SARS-CoV-2 in the nose and trachea (S. Wang et al. 2022). In human trials, UB-612 was tested for safety and immunogenicity in >4,000 subjects aged 16–85 years. The vaccine was well tolerated and had no product-related serious adverse reactions. UB-612 stimulated a robust and long-lived antibody response (>180 days) capable of neutralizing multiple, including Delta and Omicron (C.Y. Wang et al. 2022).

UB-612 was compared against three approved vaccine platforms: mRNA (Pfizer-BioNTech's Comirnaty/BNT162b2), adenovirus vector (AstraZeneca's Vaxzevria/ChAdOx1-S), and inactivated virus (Sinopharm's BIBP) in Phase 3, international, randomized, active-controlled, head-to-head heterologous booster trial. UB-612 had higher nAb titers and seroconversion rates for Omicron BA.5 and Wuhan variants than vaccines using the adenovirus vector (Vaxzevria/ChAdOx1-S) and inactivated (BIBP) platforms and was comparable to the mRNA (Comirnaty/BNT162b2) platform. UB-612 was generally safe and well tolerated. The trial recruited 944 participants across seven centers in Panama, the Philippines, and the US (Guirakhoo et al. 2022).

Vaxxinity has applied for market authorization of UB-612 in Australia and the UK (via the Provisional Registration Pathway [accelerated review] by the Therapeutic Goods Administration).

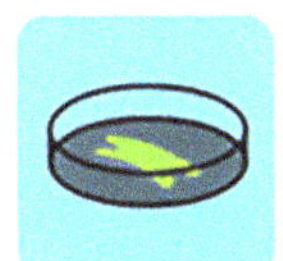

## 3.  Vaccine Pipeline

Vaxxinity's pipeline of vaccines are in different stages of preclinical and clinical trials (Table 14).

### Table 14: Vaccine Pipeline for Vaxxinity

| Vaccine Name | Indication Group | Development Stage | | | | | |
| --- | --- | --- | --- | --- | --- | --- | --- |
| | | Discovery | Preclinical | Phase 1 | Phase 2 | Phase 3 | Registration |
| UB-311 | Alzheimer's | | | | | | |
| UB-312 | Parkinson's + DLB + MSA | | | | | | |
| Tau | Alzheimer's + Other | | | | | | |
| UB-313 | Migraine | | | | | | |
| VXX-401 | Cholesterol | | | | | | |
| UB-612 | COVID-19 | | | | | | |

COVID-19 = coronavirus disease, DLB = Dementia with Lewy bodies, MSA = multiple system atrophy.

Source: Vaxxinity.

# Novel Expression Systems for Vaccine Development

Several new vaccine production methods are being employed to develop new coronavirus disease (COVID-19) vaccines. A brief explanation of the potential advantages and the challenges of these novel methods is provided in Table A1.

## Table A1:  New Expression Systems for Developing Vaccines

| System | Advantages | Challenges |
|---|---|---|
| Nucleic acid-based expression systems | RNA and DNA vaccine technologies have the potential to facilitate fast, scalable, uniform vaccine production.[a]<br><br>These vaccines use antigen-encoding nucleic acids to induce humoral and cellular immunity through specific delivery systems that enable cells to take up and express the encoded antigen. This technology can act on intracellular and extracellular targets and express a variety of proteins without entering the nucleus and without requiring in vitro expression and purification.<br><br>The development of these vaccines requires only the replacement of the antigen sequence on a mature technology platform. This may have greater agility in rapidly responding to widespread public health emergencies.<br><br>Nucleic acid-based therapeutics like RNA and DNA medicines can potentially provide new treatment options for genetic conditions that are not effectively managed with conventional medicines.[b] | Although nucleic acids can elicit robust immune responses, they are rapidly broken down by enzymes in the body. Therefore, to work, vaccines and therapeutics using this technology must be conveyed to the right cells via special delivery systems.[c]<br><br>There are two common technologies used to do this: either a virus is employed to deliver the nucleic acids (viral vector) or the nucleic acids are encapsulated in lipids.<br><br>These technologies, however, have led to several forms of harm, including hepatotoxicity, detrimental immune responses, and mutations of the recipient's DNA.<br><br>Viral vectors may stimulate the immune system to produce antibodies that attack the vector leading to a diminishing effectiveness of therapy with each dose.[d] |
| Plant-based expression systems | Plant-based expression systems potentially offer several advantages compared to conventional systems for manufacturing vaccines, diagnostics, and biopharmaceuticals (e.g., immunoglobulins, enzymes, and growth factors).[e] These include speed, flexibility and scalability of production, and safety (because they do not use animal pathogens).[f] Avoiding the use of animal products may be relevant to countries with Muslim populations.<br><br>Plant-based expression systems have been used to produce vaccine candidates and monoclonal antibodies for COVID-19, Ebola disease, HIV/AIDS, and influenza that are already being used in preclinical and clinical settings.[g] | Traditionally, recombinant proteins have been manufactured via bacterial fermentation or mammalian cell cultures. These are costly manufacturing processes, prone to contamination with pathogens, and the end products may not be highly effective at stimulating the immune system.[h] |

DNA = deoxyribonucleic acid, RNA = ribonucleic acid.

[a]  S.S. Rosa et al. 2021. mRNA Vaccines Manufacturing: Challenges and Bottlenecks. *Vaccine*. 39. pp. 2190–2200.

[b]  M.M. Silveira et al. 2021. DNA Vaccines Against COVID-19: Perspectives and Challenges. *Life Sciences*. 267. p. 118919.

[c]  G. Chen et al. 2022. Advances in the Polymeric Delivery of Nucleic Acid Vaccines. *Theranostics*. 12. pp. 4081–109.

[d]  J.L. Shirley et al. 2020. Immune Responses to Viral Gene Therapy Vectors. *Molecular Therapy*. 28(3). pp. 709–722.

[e]  B. Shanmugaraj et al. 2020. Plant Molecular Farming: A Viable Platform for Recombinant Biopharmaceutical Production. *Plants* (Basel). 9. p. 842.

[f]  B. Shanmugaraj et al. 2022. Preclinical Evaluation of a Plant-Derived SARS-Cov-2 Subunit Vaccine: Protective Efficacy, Immunogenicity, Safety, and Toxicity. *Vaccine*. 40. pp. 4440–4452.

[g]  B. Shanmugaraj et al. 2021. Potential for Developing Plant-Derived Candidate Vaccines and Biologics against Emerging Coronavirus Infections. *Pathogens*. 10. p. 1051.

[h]  B. Shanmugaraj et al. 2020. Plant Molecular Farming: A Viable Platform for Recombinant Biopharmaceutical Production. *Plants* (Basel). 9. p. 842.

Source: Asian Development Bank.

# References


J. Arya et al. 2016. Microneedle Patches for Vaccination in Developing Countries. *J Control Release*. 240. pp. 135–141.

A.V. Ballering et al. 2022. Persistence of Somatic Symptoms after COVID-19 in the Netherlands: An Observational Cohort Study. *The Lancet*. 400. pp. 452–461.

D. Balmforth et al. 2022. Evaluating the Efficacy and Safety of a Novel Prophylactic Nasal Spray in the Prevention of SARS-CoV-2 Infection: A Multi-Centre, Double Blind, Placebo-Controlled, Randomised Trial. *Journal of Clinical Virology*. 155. p. 105248.

L. Barrios et al. 2022. An Evaluation of the Safety and Immunogenicity of MVC-COV1901: Results of an Interim Analysis of a Phase III, Parallel Group, Randomized, Double-Blind, Active-Controlled Study. *medRxiv*. 14 July.

H. Bastian. 2022. And Then There Were 33…The Latest 11 Covid Vaccines to Reach the Phase 3 Results Milestone. https://absolutelymaybe.plos.org/2022/08/05/and-then-there-were-30-the-latest-9-covid-vaccines-to-reach-the-phase-3-results-milestone/.

N. Bezay et al. 2016. Safety, Immunogenicity and Dose Response of VLA84, a New Vaccine Candidate Against *Clostridium difficile*, in Healthy Volunteers. *Vaccine*. 34. pp. 2585–2592.

Biological E. 2022. Corbevax Gets DCGI Nod as a Heterologous COVID-19 Booster. https://biologicale.com/news.html

BioPharmaAPAC. 2021. Medigen's MVC-COV1901 Selected for WHO COVID-19 Solidarity Trial Vaccines. https://biopharmaapac.com/news/93/894/medigens-mvc-cov1901-selected-for-who-covid-19-solidarity-trial-vaccines.html.

C. Chen et al. 2022. Global Prevalence of Post COVID-19 Condition or Long COVID: A Meta-Analysis and Systematic Review. *The Journal of Infectious Diseases*. 226. pp. 1593–1607.

G. Chen et al. 2022. Advances in the Polymeric Delivery of Nucleic Acid Vaccines. *Theranostics*. 12. pp. 4081–4109.

J. Chen et al. 2022. A Live Attenuated Virus-Based Intranasal COVID-19 Vaccine Provides Rapid, Prolonged, and Broad Protection Against SARS-CoV-2. *Science Bulletin*. 67. pp. 1372–1387.

S.H. Cheng et al. 2021. Safety and Immunogenicity of SARS-CoV-2 S-2P Protein Vaccine MVC-COV1901 in People Living with HIV. *medRxiv*. 10 December.

A. Cherukuri et al. 2013. Adults 65 Years Old and Older Have Reduced Numbers of Functional Memory T Cells to Respiratory Syncytial Virus Fusion Protein. *Clinical and Vaccine Immunology.* 20. pp. 239–247.

C.H. Chuang et al. 2022. Titers and Breadth of Neutralizing Antibodies Against SARS-Cov-2 Variants after Heterologous Booster Vaccination in Health Care Workers Primed with Two Doses of ChAdOx1 nCov-19: A Single-Blinded, Randomized Clinical Trial. *Journal of Clinical Virology.* 157. p. 105328.

*CISION PR Newswire.* 2020. Codagenix and Serum Institute of India Announce Commencement of First-in-Human Trial of COVI-VAC, A Single Dose, Intranasal Live Attenuated Vaccine for COVID-19. https://www.prnewswire.com/news-releases/codagenix-and-serum-institute-of-india-announce-commencement-of-first-in-human-trial-of-covi-vac-a-single-dose-intranasal-live-attenuated-vaccine--for-covid-19-301191756.html.

*Codagenix.* 2022a. Codagenix Announces Award with the US Department of Defense for Development of Balanced, Tetravalent Dengue Vaccine. https://codagenix.com/codagenix-announces-award-with-the-us-department-of-defense-for-development-of-balanced-tetravalent-dengue-vaccine/.

*Codagenix.* 2022b. Codagenix Intranasal COVID-19 Vaccine Shows Potent Cellular Immune Response Against Conserved Viral Proteins, Indicating Potential for Immunogenicity Against Omicron and Future Variants in Phase 1 Data. https://codagenix.com/codagenix-intranasal-covid-19-vaccine-shows-potent-cellular-immune-response-against-conserved-viral-proteins-indicating-potential-for-immunogenicity-against-omicron-and-future-variants-in-phase-1-dat/.

J.R. Coleman et al. 2008. Virus Attenuation by Genome-Scale Changes in Codon Pair Bias. *Science.* 320. pp. 1784–1787.

P. Comstedt et al. 2014. Design and Development of a Novel Vaccine for Protection Against Lyme Borreliosis. *PloS One.* 9. p. e113294.

P. Comstedt et al. 2015. Characterization and Optimization of a Novel Vaccine for Protection Against Lyme Borreliosis. *Vaccine.* 33. pp. 5982–5988.

P. Comstedt et al. 2017. The Novel Lyme Borreliosis Vaccine VLA15 Shows Broad Protection Against Borrelia Species Expressing Six Different Ospa Serotypes. *PloS One.* 12. p. e0184357.

J.P. Cramer et al. 2016. Immunogenicity and Safety of the Inactivated Japanese Encephalitis Vaccine IXIARO® in Elderly Subjects: Open-Label, Uncontrolled, Multi-center, Phase 4 Study. *Vaccine.* 34. pp. 4579–4585.

C. Davies et al. 2022. Usability, Acceptability, and Feasibility of a High-Density Microarray Patch (HD-MAP) Applicator as a Delivery Method for Vaccination in Clinical Settings. *Human Vaccines & Immunotherapeutics.* 18. p. 2018863.

R. de Alwis et al. 2021. A Single Dose of Self-Transcribing and Replicating RNA-Based SARS-CoV-2 Vaccine Produces Protective Adaptive Immunity in Mice. *Molecular Therapy: The Journal of the American Society of Gene Therapy.* 29. pp. 1970–1983.

L.M. de la Maza, T.L. Darville, and S. Pal. 2021. Chlamydia Trachomatis Vaccines for Genital Infections: Where Are We and How Far Is There to Go? *Expert Review of Vaccines.* 20. pp. 421–435.

Developing Countries Vaccine Manufacturers Network. *New HPV Vaccine from Innovax Receives WHO Prequalification.* https://dcvmn.org/New-HPV-vaccine-from-Innovax-receives-WHO-Prequalification/.

P. Devnath et al. 2022. The Pathogenesis of Nipah Virus: A Review. *Microbial Pathogenesis.* 170. p. 105693.

R. Diaz-Trelles et al. 2022. Lipid Nanoparticle Delivers Phenylalanine Ammonia Lyase mRNA to the Liver Leading to Catabolism and Clearance of Phenylalanine in a Phenylketonuria Mouse Model. *Molecular Genetics and Metabolism Reports.* 32. p. 100882.

K. Dubischar-Kastner et al. 2010a. Long-Term Immunity and Immune Response to a Booster Dose Following Vaccination with the Inactivated Japanese Encephalitis Vaccine IXIARO, IC51. *Vaccine.* 28. pp. 5197–5202.

K. Dubischar-Kastner et al. 2010b. Safety Analysis of a Vero-Cell Culture Derived Japanese Encephalitis Vaccine, IXIARO® (IC51), in 6 Months of Follow-up. *Vaccine.* 28. pp. 6463–6469.

K.L. Dubischar et al. 2017a. Immunogenicity of the Inactivated Japanese Encephalitis Virus Vaccine IXIARO in Children from a Japanese Encephalitis Virus-endemic Region. *The Pediatric Infectious Disease Journal.* 36. pp. 898–904.

K.L. Dubischar et al. 2017b. Safety of the Inactivated Japanese Encephalitis Virus Vaccine IXIARO in Children: An Open-label, Randomized, Active-Controlled, Phase 3 Study. *Pediatric Infectious Disease Journal.* 36. pp. 889–897.

S. Eder et al. 2011. Long Term Immunity Following a Booster Dose of the Inactivated Japanese Encephalitis Vaccine IXIARO®, IC51. *Vaccine.* 29. pp. 2607–2612.

J.H. Erasmus et al. 2020. An *Alphavirus*-Derived Replicon RNA Vaccine Induces SARS-Cov-2 Neutralizing Antibody and T Cell Responses in Mice and Nonhuman Primates. *Science Translational Medicine.* 12. p. eabc9396.

K. Esser-Nobis et al. 2020. Spatiotemporal Dynamics of Innate Immune Signaling via RIG-I-like Receptors. *PNAS.* 117. pp. 15778–15788.

J.A. Estrada et al. 2022. An Immunobridging Study to Evaluate the Neutralizing Antibody Titer in Adults Immunized with Two Doses of Either ChAdOx1-nCov-19 (AstraZeneca) or MVC-COV1901. *Vaccines (Basel).* 10. p. 655.

European Medicines Agency. 2022a. *EMA Recommends Approval of VidPrevtyn Beta as a COVID-19 Booster Vaccine.* https://www.ema.europa.eu/en/news/ema-recommends-approval-vidprevtyn-beta-covid-19-booster-vaccine.

European Medicines Agency. 2022b. *EMA Recommends Valneva's COVID-19 Vaccine for Authorisation in the EU.* https://www.ema.europa.eu/en/news/ema-recommends-valnevas-covid-19-vaccine-authorisation-eu.

European Medicines Agency. 2022c. *Ixiaro.* https://www.ema.europa.eu/en/medicines/human/EPAR/ixiaro.

European Medicines Agency. *PRIME: Priority Medicines*. https://www.ema.europa.eu/en/human-regulatory/research-development/prime-priority-medicines.

A. Forster and M. Junger. 2022. Opportunities and Challenges for Commercializing Microarray Patches for Vaccination from a MAP Developer's Perspective. *Human Vaccines & Immunotherapeutics*. 18. p. 2050123.

A.H. Forster et al. 2020. Safety, Tolerability, and Immunogenicity of Influenza Vaccination with a High-Density Microarray Patch: Results from a Randomized, Controlled Phase I Clinical Trial. *PloS Med*. 17. p. e1003024.

J.R. Francica et al. 2021. Protective Antibodies Elicited by SARS-Cov-2 Spike Protein Vaccination Are Boosted in the Lung after Challenge in Nonhuman Primates. *Science Translational Medicine*. 13. p. eabi4547.

P. Fuentes-Prior et al. 2021. Priming of SARS-CoV-2 S Protein by Several Membrane-Bound Serine Proteinases Could Explain Enhanced Viral Infectivity and Systemic COVID-19 Infection. *The Journal of Biological Chemistry*. 29. p. 100135.

D.H. Fuller and P. Berglund. 2020. Amplifying RNA Vaccine Development. *NEJM*. 382. pp. 2469–2471.

O. Gholizadeh et al. 2022. Recent Advances in Treatment Crimean-Congo Hemorrhagic Fever Virus: A Concise Overview. *Microbial Pathogenesis*. 169. p. 105657.

P.A. Goepfert et al. 2021. Safety and Immunogenicity of SARS-Cov-2 Recombinant Protein Vaccine Formulations in Healthy Adults: Interim Results of a Randomised, Placebo-Controlled, Phase 1-2, Dose-Ranging Study. *Lancet Infectious Diseases*. 21. pp. 1257–1270.

Government of Australia, Department of Health and Aged Care. *Flublok Quadrivalent*. https://www.tga.gov.au/resources/auspmd/flublok-quadrivalent.

F. Guirakhoo et al. 2022. High Neutralizing Antibody Levels Against Severe Acute Respiratory Syndrome Coronavirus 2 Omicron BA.1 and BA.2 After UB-612 Vaccine Booster. *The Journal of Infectious Diseases*. 226. pp. 1401–1406.

S. Guzmán-López et al. 2022. Clinical and Immunologic Efficacy of the Recombinant Adenovirus Type-5-Vectored (CanSino Bio) Vaccine in University Professors during the COVID-19 Delta Wave. *Vaccines (Basel)*. 10 (5). p. 656.

S.A. Halperin et al. 2022. Final Efficacy Analysis, Interim Safety Analysis, and Immunogenicity of a Single Dose of Recombinant Novel Coronavirus Vaccine (Adenovirus Type 5 Vector) in Adults 18 Years and Older: An International, Multicentre, Randomised, Double-Blinded, Placebo-Controlled Phase 3 Trial. *The Lancet*. 399. pp. 237–248.

M. Hashimoto et al. 2022. Immunogenicity and Protective Efficacy of SARS-CoV-2 Recombinant S-protein Vaccine S-268019-B in Cynomolgus Monkeys. *Vaccine*. 40. pp. 4231–41.

*Hindustan Times*. 2022. Biological E. Cuts Price of Corbevax COVID-19 Vaccine to ₹250 per Dose. https://www.hindustantimes.com/business/biological-e-cuts-price-of-corbevax-covid-19-vaccine-to-250-per-dose-101652689615837.html.

S.M. Hsieh et al. 2021a. *The Lancet Respiratory Medicine.* 9. pp. 1396–1406.

S.M. Hsieh et al. 2021b. Safety and Immunogenicity of a Recombinant Stabilized Prefusion SARS-CoV-2 Spike Protein Vaccine (MVCCOV1901) Adjuvanted with CpG 1018 and Aluminum Hydroxide in Healthy Adults: A Phase 1, Dose-Escalation Study. *eClinicalMedicine* 38. p. 100989.

S.M. Hsieh et al. 2022. *medRxiv.* 4 January.

L. M. Huang et al. 2019. *Vaccine.* 37. pp. 1827–1835.

A. Impagliazzo et al. 2015. A Stable Trimeric Influenza Hemagglutinin Stem as a Broadly Protective Immunogen. *Science.* 349. pp. 1301–1306.

*India Today*. 2022. Corbevax Safe for Kids, Offers High Antibody Levels, Says Biological E CEO EXCLUSIVE. https://www.indiatoday.in/coronavirus-outbreak/vaccine-updates/story/corbevax-safe-for-kids-offers-high-antibody-levels-says-biological-e-ceo-1926215-2022-03-16.

S. Iwata et al. 2022. Phase 1/2 Clinical Trial Of COVID-19 Vaccine in Japanese Participants: A Report of Interim Findings. *Vaccine.* 40. pp. 3721–3726.

T. Jelinek et al. 2018.  Safety and Immunogenicity of an Inactivated Vero Cell_Derived Japanese Encephalitis Vaccine (IXIARO, JESPECT) in a Pediatric Population in JE Non-endemic Countries: An Uncontrolled, Open-Label Phase 3 Study. *Travel Medicine and Infectious Disease.* 22. pp. 18–24.

L. Jin et al. 2022. Antibody Persistence and Safety through 6 Months after Heterologous Orally Aerosolised Ad5-nCoV in Individuals Primed with  T w o - D o s e  CoronaVac Previously. *medRxiv.* 28 July.

V. Kadlecek et al. 2018. Antibody Persistence up to 3 Years after Primary Immunization with Inactivated Japanese Encephalitis Vaccine IXIARO in Philippine Children and Effect of a Booster Dose. *Pediatric Infectious Disease Journal.* 37. pp. e233–e240.

A. Kaltenbock et al. 2009. Safety and Immunogenicity of Concomitant Vaccination with the Cell-Culture Based Japanese Encephalitis Vaccine IC51 and the Hepatitis A Vaccine HAVRIX 1440 in Healthy Subjects: A Single-Blind, Randomized, Controlled Phase 3 Study. *Vaccine.* 27. pp. 4483–4489.

A. Kaltenbock et al. 2010. Immunogenicity and Safety of IXIARO (IC51) in a Phase II Study in Healthy Indian Children Between 1 and 3 Years of Age. *Vaccine.* 28. pp. 834–839.

N. Khorattanakulchai et al. 2022a. A Recombinant Subunit Vaccine Candidate Produced in Plants Elicits Neutralizing Antibodies Against SARS-CoV-2 Variants in Macaques. *Frontiers in Plant Science.* 13. p. 901978.

N. Khorattanakulchai et al. 2022b. Receptor Binding Domain Proteins of SARS-CoV-2 Variants Produced in *Nicotiana benthamiana* Elicit Neutralizing Antibodies Against Variants of Concern. *Journal of Medical Virology.* 94. pp. 4265–4276.

H. Kollaritsch, M. Paulke-Korinek, and K. Dubischar-Kastner. 2009. Japanese Encephalitis Vaccine. *Expert Opinion on Biological Therapy.* 9. pp. 921–931.

T.Y. Kuo et al. 2020. Development of CpG-Adjuvanted Stable Prefusion SARS-CoV-2 Spike Antigen as a Subunit Vaccine Against COVID-19. *Scientific Reports.* 10. p. 20085.

T.Y. Kuo et al. 2022a. Hamsters Protected from SARS-CoV-2 Delta Variant Challenge after Two Doses of Adjuvanted SARS-CoV-2 Recombinant Spike Protein (S-2P) and One Dose of Beta S-2P. *The Journal of Infectious Diseases.* 226. pp. 1562–1567.

T.Y. Kuo et al. 2022b. Neutralization of SARS-CoV-2 Omicron BA.4/BA.5 Subvariant by a Booster Dose of Bivalent Adjuvanted Subunit Vaccine Containing Omicron BA.4/BA.5 and BA.1 Subvariants. *bioRxiv.*

*The Lancet.* 2018. GLOBOCAN 2018: Counting the Toll of Cancer. *The Lancet.* 392 (10152). p. 985.

R. Lazarus et al. 2022a. Immunogenicity and Safety of an Inactivated Whole-Virus COVID-19 Vaccine (VLA2001) Compared with the Adenoviral Vector Vaccine ChAdOx1-S in Adults in the UK (COV-COMPARE): Interim Analysis of a Randomised, Controlled, Phase 3, Immunobridging Trial. *Lancet Infectious Diseases.* 22. pp. 1716–1727.

R. Lazarus et al. 2022b. Safety and Immunogenicity of the Inactivated Whole-Virus Adjuvanted COVID-19 Vaccine VLA2001: A Randomized, Dose Escalation, Double-Blind Phase 1/2 Clinical Trial in Healthy Adults. *The Journal of Infection.* 85. pp. 306–317.

C. Le Nouën et al. 2017. Genetic Stability of Genome-Scale Deoptimized RNA Virus Vaccine Candidates under Selective Pressure. *Proceedings of the National Academy of Sciences.* 114(3). pp. E386-E395.

S. Lee et al. 2021. Suppression of Hepatitis B Virus Through Therapeutic Activation of RIG-I and IRF3 Signaling in Hepatocytes. *iScience* 24. p. 101969.

J.X. Li et al. 2017. Immunity Duration of a Recombinant Adenovirus Type-5 Vector-Based Ebola Vaccine and a Homologous Prime-Boost Immunisation in Healthy Adults in People's Republic of China: Final Report of a Randomised, Double-Blind, Placebo-Controlled, Phase 1 Trial. *The Lancet Global Health.* 5. pp. e324–e334.

J.X. Li et al. 2022. Safety and Immunogenicity of Heterologous Boost Immunisation with an Orally Administered Aerosolised Ad5-nCoV after Two-Dose Priming with an Inactivated SARS-CoV-2 Vaccine in Chinese Adults: A Randomised, Open-Label, Single-Centre Trial. *The Lancet Respiratory Medicine.* 10. pp. 739–478.

M.L. Li et al. 2021. Enterovirus A71 Vaccines. *Vaccines (Basel).* 9. p. 199.

Y. Li et al. 2018. Establishing China's National Standard for the Recombinant Adenovirus Type 5 Vector-Based Ebola Vaccine (Ad5-EBOV) Virus Titer. *Human Gene Therapy. Clinical Development.* 29. pp. 226–232.

Y. Li et al. 2022. Global, Regional, and National Disease Burden Estimates of Acute Lower Respiratory Infections Due to Respiratory Syncytial Virus in Children Younger Than 5 Years in 2019: A Systematic Analysis. *The Lancet.* 399. pp. 2047–2064.

Z.P. Li et al. 2022. Batch-to-Batch Consistency Trial of an Adenovirus Type-5 Vector-Based COVID-19 Vaccine in Adults Aged 18 Years and Above. *Expert Review of Vaccines.* pp. 1843–1849.

C.E. Lien et al. 2021. CpG-Adjuvanted Stable Prefusion SARS-CoV-2 Spike Protein Protected Hamsters from SARS-CoV-2 Challenge. *Scientific Reports.* 11. p. 8761.

C.E. Lien et al. 2022. Evaluating the Neutralizing Ability of a CpG-Adjuvanted S-2P Subunit Vaccine Against Severe Acute Respiratory Syndrome Coronavirus 2 (SARS-CoV-2) Variants of Concern. *Clinical Infectious Diseases: An Official Publication of the Infectious Diseases Society of America.* 74. pp. 1899–1905.

Y. Lin et al. 2022. Protection of Hamsters Challenged with SARS-CoV-2 After Two Doses of MVC-COV1901 Vaccine Followed by a Single Intranasal Booster with Nanoemulsion Adjuvanted S-2P Vaccine. *Scientific Reports.* 12. p. 11369.

J. Liu et al. 2022. Preclinical Evaluation of a SARS-CoV-2 mRNA Vaccine PTX-COVID19-B. *Science Advances.* 8. p. eabj9815.

K. Lundstrom et al. 2021. Self-Replicating RNA Viruses for Vaccine Development Against Infectious Diseases and Cancer. 2021. *Vaccines (Basel).* 9. p. 1187.

E. Mahase et al. 2022. UK Approves Valneva Vaccine for Adults under 50. *BMJ.* 377. p. o985.

G. Maki and M. Zervos. 2021. Health Care-Acquired Infections in Low- and Middle-Income Countries and the Role of Infection Prevention and Control. *Infectious Disease Clinics of North America.* 35. pp. 827–39.

C.L.D. McMillan et al. 2021. Complete Protection by a Single-Dose Skin Patch-Delivered SARS-CoV-2 Spike Vaccine. *Science Advances.* 7. p. eabj8065.

E.M. Mucker et al. 2020. Lipid Nanoparticle Formulation Increases Efficiency of DNA-Vectored Vaccines/Immunoprophylaxis in Animals Including Transchromosomic Bovines. *Scientific Reports.* 10. p. 8764.

S. Mueller et al. 2020. A Codon-Pair Deoptimized Live-Attenuated Vaccine Against Respiratory Syncytial Virus is Immunogenic and Efficacious in Non-human Primates. *Vaccine.* 38. pp. 2943–2948.

D.A. Muller et al. 2020. Innate Local Response and Tissue Recovery Following Application of High Density Microarray Patches to Human Skin. *Scientific Reports.* 10. p. 18468.

A.P.S. Munro et al. 2021. Safety and Immunogenicity of Seven COVID-19 Vaccines as a Third Dose (Booster) Following Two Doses of ChAdOx1 nCov-19 or BNT162b2 in the UK (COV-BOOST): A Blinded, Multicentre, Randomised, Controlled, Phase 2 Trial. *The Lancet.* 398. pp. 2258–2276.

S. Nasreen et al. 2022. Effectiveness of COVID-19 Vaccines Against Symptomatic SARS-CoV-2 Infection and Severe Outcomes with Variants of Concern in Ontario. *Nature Microbiology.* 7. pp. 379–385.

T.P. Nguyen et al. 2022a. Safety and Immunogenicity of Nanocovax, a SARS-CoV-2 Recombinant Spike Protein Vaccine: Interim Results of a Double-Blind, Randomised Controlled Phase 1 and 2 Trial. *The Lancet Regional Health. Western Pacific.* 24. p. 100474.

T.P. Nguyen et al. 2022b. The Efficacy, Safety and Immunogenicity Nanocovax: Results of a Randomized, Double-Blind, Placebo-Controlled Phase 3 Trial. *medRxiv.* 23 March.

T.T. Nguyen et al. 2022. Efficacy, Safety, and Immunogenicity of an Inactivated, Adjuvanted Enterovirus 71 Vaccine in Infants and Children: A Multiregion, Double-Blind, Randomised, Placebo-Controlled, Phase 3 Trial. *The Lancet.* 399. pp. 1708–1717.

N.M. Orozco et al. 2022. Phase I Study of a SARS-CoV-2 mRNA Vaccine PTX-COVID19-B. *medRxiv.* 10 May.

C. Panapitakkul et al. 2022. Plant-Produced S1 Subunit Protein of SARS-CoV-2 Elicits Immunogenic Responses in Mice. *Vaccines (Basel).* 10. p. 1961.

D.M. Parkin et al. 2005. Global Cancer Statistics, 2002. *CA: A Cancer Journal for Clinicians.* 55. pp. 74–108.

M. Parrish. 2022. *Vaxxinity Looks to Pioneer the Next Revolution in Pharma.* https://www.pharmavoice.com/news/vaxxinity-to-pioneer-the-next-revolution/617229/.

M. Pastor, J.L. Pedraz, and A. Esquisabel. 2013. The State-of-the-Art of Approved and Under-development Cholera Vaccines. *Vaccine.* 31. pp. 4069–4078.

Pharmaceutical Technology. 2022. *HDT Bio Receives Emergency Use Approval for Covid-19 Vaccine in India.* https://www.pharmaceutical-technology.com/news/hdt-bio-vaccine-india-approval/.

V. Pavot et al. 2022. Protein-Based SARS-CoV-2 Spike Vaccine Booster Increases Cross-Neutralization Against SARS-Cov-2 Variants of Concern in Non-Human Primates. *Nature Communications.* 13. p. 1699.

F.E. Pearson et al. 2013. Dry-Coated Live Viral Vector Vaccines Delivered by Nanopatch Microprojections Retain Long-Term Thermostability and Induce Transgene-Specific T Cell Responses in Mice. *PLoS One.* 8. p. e67888.

Y. Pei et al. 2022. Synthesis and Bioactivity of Readily Hydrolysable Novel Cationic Lipids for Potential Lung Delivery Application of mRNAs. *Chemistry and Physics of Lipids.* 243. p. 105178.

C.G. Perez-Garcia et al. 2022. Development of an mRNA Replacement Therapy for Phenylketonuria. *Molecular Therapy. Nucleic Acids.* 28. pp. 87–98.

J. Pollet et al. 2022. Receptor-Binding Domain Recombinant Protein on Alum-CpG Induces Broad Protection Against SARS-CoV-2 Variants of Concern. *Vaccine.* 40. pp. 3655–3663.

A. Poudel et al. 2019. Access to Palliative Care: Discrepancy Among Low-Income and High-Income Countries. *Journal of Global Health.* 9. p. 020309.

T.W. Prow et al. 2010. Nanopatch-Targeted Skin Vaccination Against West Nile Virus and Chikungunya Virus in Mice. *Small.* 6. pp. 1776–1784.

Y.L. Qiao et al. 2020. Efficacy, Safety, and Immunogenicity of an *Escherichia coli*-Produced Bivalent Human Papillomavirus Vaccine: An Interim Analysis of a Randomized Clinical Trial. *Journal of the National Cancer Institute.* 112. pp. 145–153.

S. Ramaswamy et al. 2017. Systemic Delivery of Factor IX Messenger RNA for Protein Replacement Therapy. *PNAS.* 114. pp. E1941–E1950.

*Reuters*. 2022. Australia's CSL in mRNA Vaccine Licensing Deal with U.S.-Based Arcturus. https://www.reuters
.com/business/healthcare-pharmaceuticals/australias-csl-mrna-vaccine-licensing-deal-with-arcturus
-2022-11-01/.

V.L. Richardson et al. 2022. Vaccine Effectiveness of CanSino (Adv5-nCoV) Coronavirus Disease 2019
(COVID-19) Vaccine Among Childcare Workers—Mexico, March–December 2021. *Clinical Infectious
Diseases: An Official Publication of the Infectious Diseases Society of America.* 75 (Supplement 2).
pp. S167–S173.

G.V.T. Roozen et al. 2022. COVID-19 Vaccine Dose Sparing: Strategies to Improve Vaccine Equity and Pandemic
Preparedness. *The Lancet Global Health.* 10. pp. e570–e573.

P. Roques et al. 2017. Attenuated and Vectored Vaccines Protect Nonhuman Primates Against Chikungunya
Virus. *Journal of Clinical Investigation Insight.* 2. p. e83527.

S.S. Rosa et al. 2021. mRNA Vaccines Manufacturing: Challenges and Bottlenecks. *Vaccine.* 39. pp. 2190–2200.

R. Schlegl et al. 2015. *Vaccine.* 33. pp. 5989–5996.

E. Schuller et al. 2008a. Effect of Pre-existing Anti-Tick-Borne Encephalitis Virus Immunity on Neutralising
Antibody Response to the Vero Cell-Derived, Inactivated Japanese Encephalitis Virus Vaccine Candidate
IC51. *Vaccine.* 26. pp. 6151–6156.

E. Schuller et al. 2008b. Long-Term Immunogenicity of the New Vero Cell-Derived, Inactivated Japanese
Encephalitis Virus Vaccine IC51: Six and 12 Month Results of a Multicenter Follow-up Phase 3 Study.
*Vaccine.* 26. pp. 4382–4386.

E. Schuller et al. 2009. Comparison of a Single, High-Dose Vaccination Regimen to the Standard Regimen for the
Investigational Japanese Encephalitis Vaccine, IC51: A Randomized, Observer-Blind, Controlled Phase 3
Study. *Vaccine.* 27. pp. 2188–2193.

E. Schuller et al. 2011. Safety Profile of the Vero Cell-Derived Japanese Encephalitis Virus (JEV) Vaccine IXIARO.
*Vaccine.* 29. pp. 8669–8676.

H. Shaikh et al. 2020. Current and Future Cholera Vaccines. *Vaccine.* 38 (Suppl 1). pp. A118–A126.

B. Shanmugaraj et al. 2020. Plant Molecular Farming: A Viable Platform for Recombinant Biopharmaceutical
Production. *Plants (Basel).* 9. p. 842.

B. Shanmugaraj et al. 2021. Potential for Developing Plant-Derived Candidate Vaccines and Biologics against
Emerging Coronavirus Infections. *Pathogens.* 10. p. 1051.

B. Shanmugaraj et al. 2022. Preclinical Evaluation of a Plant-Derived SARS-Cov-2 Subunit Vaccine: Protective
Efficacy, Immunogenicity, Safety, and Toxicity. *Vaccine.* 40. pp. 4440–4452.

M. Shinkai et al. 2022. Immunogenicity and Safety of Booster Dose of S-268019-B or BNT162b2 in Japanese
Participants: An Interim Report of Phase 2/3, Randomized, Observer-Blinded, Noninferiority Study. *Vaccine*
40. pp. 4328–4333.

Shionogi. 2022. Shionogi Files for Approval of S-268019, a COVID-19 Recombinant Protein-Based Vaccine, in Japan. https://www.shionogi.com/global/en/news/2022/11/2022112401.html.

J.L. Shirley et al. 2020. Immune Responses to Viral Gene Therapy Vectors. *Molecular Therapy: The Journal of the American Society of Gene Therapy*. 28. pp. 709–722.

L.A. Silva and T.S. Dermody. 2017. Chikungunya Virus: Epidemiology, Replication, Disease Mechanisms, and Prospective Intervention Strategies. *The Journal of Clinical Investigation*. 127. pp. 737–749.

M.M. Silveira et al. 2021. DNA Vaccines Against COVID-19: Perspectives and Challenges. *Life Sciences*. 267. p. 118919.

K. Siriwattananon et al. 2021. Immunogenicity Studies of Plant-Produced SARS-CoV-2 Receptor Binding Domain-Based Subunit Vaccine Candidate with Different Adjuvant Formulations. *Vaccines (Basel)*. 9. p. 744.

J.S. Solís Arce et al. 2021. COVID-19 Vaccine Acceptance and Hesitancy in Low- and Middle-Income Countries. *Nature Medicine*. 27. pp. 1385–1394.

S. Sridhar et al. 2022. Safety and Immunogenicity of an AS03-Adjuvanted SARS-Cov-2 Recombinant Protein Vaccine (CoV2 preS dTM) in Healthy Adults: Interim Findings from a Phase 2, Randomised, Dose-Finding, Multicentre Study. *Lancet Infectious Diseases*. 22. pp. 636–648.

C.B. Stauft et al. 2018. Extensive Recoding of Dengue Virus Type 2 Specifically Reduces Replication in Primate Cells Without Gain-of-Function in *Aedes aegypti* Mosquitoes. *PLoS One*. 13. p. e0198303.

C.B. Stauft et al. 2019. Live-Attenuated H1N1 Influenza Vaccine Candidate Displays Potent Efficacy in Mice and Ferrets. *PLoS One*. 14. p. e0223784.

D. Stuckler et al. 2008. Population Causes and Consequences of Leading Chronic Diseases: A Comparative Analysis of Prevailing Explanations. *The Milbank Quarterly*. 86. pp. 273–326.

E. Tauber et al. 2007. Safety and Immunogenicity of a Vero-Cell-Derived, Inactivated Japanese Encephalitis Vaccine: A Non-inferiority, Phase III, Randomised Controlled Trial. *The Lancet*. 370. pp. 1847–1853.

E. Tauber et al. 2008. Randomized, Double-Blind, Placebo-Controlled Phase 3 Trial of the Safety and Tolerability of IC51, an Inactivated Japanese Encephalitis Vaccine. *The Journal of Infectious Diseases*. 198. pp. 493–499.

C. Taucher, H. Kollaritsch, and K.L. Dubischar. 2019. Persistence of the Immune Response after Vaccination with the Japanese Encephalitis Vaccine, IXIARO® in Healthy Adults: A Five Year Follow-up Study. *Vaccine*. 37. pp. 2529–2531.

S. Thuluva et al. 2022a. Evaluation of Safety and Immunogenicity of Receptor-Binding Domain-Based COVID-19 Vaccine (Corbevax) to Select the Optimum Formulation in Open-Label, Multicentre, and Randomised Phase-1/2 and Phase-2 Clinical Trials. *EBioMedicine*. 83. p. 104217.

S. Thuluva et al. 2022b. Safety, Tolerability and Immunogenicity of Biological E's CORBEVAX Vaccine in Children and Adolescents: A Prospective, Randomised, Double-Blind, Placebo Controlled, Phase-2/3 study. *Vaccine* 40. pp. 7130–7140.

S. Thuluva et al. 2022c. Selection of Optimum Formulation of RBD-Based Protein Sub-unit COVID-19 Vaccine (Corbevax) Based on Safety and Immunogenicity in an Open-Label, Randomized Phase-1 and 2 Clinical Studies. *medRxiv*. 16 March.

*The Times of India.* 2021. India Approves Corbevax, Covovax Vaccines for Emergency Use. https://timesofindia .indiatimes.com/india/india-approves-corbevax-covovax-vaccines-for-emergency-use/articleshow/ 88555029.cms.

T.N.M. Tran et al. 2021. Preclinical Immune Response and Safety Evaluation of the Protein Subunit Vaccine Nanocovax for COVID-19. *Frontiers in Immunology.* 12. p. 766112.

US Food and Drug Administration (FDA). *Fast Track.* https://www.fda.gov/patients/fast-track-breakthrough-therapy-accelerated-approval-priority-review/fast-track.

US FDA. *Ixiaro.* https://www.fda.gov/vaccines-blood-biologics/vaccines/ixiaro.

Valneva. *Dukoral.* https://www.valneva.co.uk/healthcare-professionals/dukoral.

A. Waits et al. 2022. Safety and Immunogenicity of MVC-COV1901 Vaccine in Older Adults: Phase 2 Randomized Dose-Comparison Trial. *International Journal of Infectious Diseases: Official Publication of the International Society for Infectious Diseases.* 124. pp. 21–26.

E. Waltz. 2022. How Nasal-Spray Vaccines Could Change the Pandemic. *Nature.* 609. pp. 240–242.

Y. Wan et al. 2021. Formulation Development and Improved Stability of a Combination Measles and Rubella Live-Viral Vaccine Dried for Use in the Nanopatch Microneedle Delivery System. *Human Vaccines & Immunotherapeutics.* 17. pp. 2501–2516.

C.Y. Wang et al. 2022. A Multitope SARS-CoV-2 Vaccine Provides Long-Lasting B Cell and T Cell Immunity Against Delta and Omicron Variants. *The Journal of Clinical Investigation.* 132. p. e157707.

H. Wang et al. 2022. mRNA Based Vaccines Provide Broad Protection Against Different SARS-CoV-2 Variants of Concern. *Emerging Microbes & Infections.* 11. pp. 1550–1553.

S. Wang et al. 2022. A Novel RBD-Protein/Peptide Vaccine Elicits Broadly Neutralizing Antibodies and Protects Mice and Macaques against SARS-CoV-2. *Emerging Microbes & Infections.* 11. pp. 2724–2734.

W. Wang et al. 2022. Development of a Skin- and Neuro-Attenuated Live Vaccine for Varicella. *Nature Communications.* 13. p. 824.

Y. Wang et al. 2021. Scalable Live-Attenuated SARS-CoV-2 Vaccine Candidate Demonstrates Preclinical Safety and Efficacy. *The Proceedings of the National Academy of Sciences.* 118. p. e2102775118.

L. Wei et al. 2021. Elimination of Cervical Cancer: Challenges Promoting the HPV Vaccine in China. *Indian Journal of Gynecologic Oncology*. 19. p. 51.

World Health Organization (WHO). 2012. *Global Vaccine Action Plan*. Geneva. https://www.who.int/teams/ immunization-vaccines-and-biologicals/strategies/global-vaccine-action-plan.

WHO. 2020. *The Top 10 Causes of Death*. Geneva. https://www.who.int/news-room/fact-sheets/detail/the-top-10-causes-of-death.

WHO. 2022. *WHO Validates 11th Vaccine for COVID-19*. https://www.who.int/news/item/19-05-2022-who-validates-11th-vaccine-for-covid-19.

N. Wressnigg et al. 2020. Single-Shot Live-Attenuated Chikungunya Vaccine in Healthy Adults: A Phase 1, Randomised Controlled Trial. *The Lancet Infectious Diseases*. 20. pp. 1193–1203.

N.V. Wressnigg et al. 2022. A Randomized, Placebo-Controlled, Blinded Phase 1 Study Investigating a Novel Inactivated, Vero Cell-Culture Derived Zika Virus Vaccine. *Journal of Travel Medicine*.

S. Wu et al. 2021. Safety, Tolerability, and Immunogenicity of an Aerosolised Adenovirus Type-5 Vector-Based COVID-19 Vaccine (Ad5-Ncov) in Adults: Preliminary Report of an Open-Label and Randomised Phase 1 Clinical Trial. *Lancet Infectious Diseases*. 21. pp. 1654–1664.

T. Wu et al. 2012. Hepatitis E Vaccine Development: A 14 Year Odyssey. *Human Vaccines & Immunotherapeutics*. 8. pp. 823–827.

Z. Xie et al. 2020. A Phase III Clinical Trial Study on the Safety and Immunogenicity of ACYW135 Group Meningococcal Conjugate Vaccine Inoculated in 3 month old Infants. *Chinese Journal of Preventative Medicine*. 54. pp. 947–952.

Z. Xie et al. 2021a. A Phase III Clinical Trial Study on the Safety and Immunogenicity of ACYW135 Group Meningococcal Conjugate Vaccine Inoculated in 3 Month Old Infants. *Chinese Journal of Vaccines and Immunization*. 27. pp. 540–546.

Z. Xie et al. 2021b. Safety of a Domestic Group A, C, Y, and W135 Meningococcal Conjugate Vaccine among 3-Month-Old, 6-23-Month-Old, and 2-6-Year-Old Children: A Phase III Clinical Trial. *Chinese Journal of Vaccines and Immunization*. 27. pp. 648–654.

F. Xu et al. 2022. Safety, Mucosal and Systemic Immunopotency of an Aerosolized Adenovirus-Vectored Vaccine Against SARS-CoV-2 in Rhesus Macaques. *Emerging Microbes & Infections*. 11. pp. 438–441.

S.M. Yoo et al. 2022. Factors Associated with Post-Acute Sequelae of SARS-CoV-2 (PASC) after Diagnosis of Symptomatic COVID-19 in the Inpatient and Outpatient Setting in a Diverse Cohort. *Journal of General Internal Medicine*. 37. pp. 1988–1995.

H. Yu et al. 2022. Restoring Ornithine Transcarbamylase (OTC) Activity in an OTC-Deficient Mouse Model Using LUNAR-OTC mRNA. *Clinical and Translational Science*. 2. p. e33.

R. Yumul et al. 2016. Epithelial Junction Opener Improves Oncolytic Adenovirus Therapy in Mouse Tumor Models. *Human Gene Therapy*. 27. pp. 325–337.

J. Zhang et al. 2015. Long-Term Efficacy of a Hepatitis E Vaccine. *The New England Journal of Medicine*. 372. pp. 914–922.

F.H. Zhao et al. 2022. Efficacy, Safety, and Immunogenicity of an *Escherichia coli*-Produced Human Papillomavirus (16 and 18) L1 Virus-Like-Particle Vaccine: End-of-Study Analysis of a Phase 3, Double-Blind, Randomised, Controlled Trial. *Lancet Infectious Diseases*. 22. pp. 1756–1768.

F.C. Zhu et al. 2010. Efficacy and Safety of a Recombinant Hepatitis E Vaccine in Healthy Adults: A Large-Scale, Randomised, Double-Blind Placebo-Controlled, Phase 3 Trial. *The Lancet*. 376. pp. 895–902.

F.C. Zhu et al. 2015. Safety and Immunogenicity of a Novel Recombinant Adenovirus Type-5 Vector-Based Ebola Vaccine in Healthy Adults in China: Preliminary Report of a Randomised, Double-Blind, Placebo-Controlled, Phase 1 Trial. *The Lancet*. 385. pp. 2272–2279.

F.C. Zhu et al. 2017. Safety and Immunogenicity of a Recombinant Adenovirus Type-5 Vector-Based Ebola Vaccine in Healthy Adults in Sierra Leone: A Single-Centre, Randomised, Double-Blind, Placebo-Controlled, Phase 2 Trial. *The Lancet*. 389. pp. 621–628.

F.C. Zhu et al. 2020a. Immunogenicity and Safety of a Recombinant Adenovirus Type-5-Vectored COVID-19 Vaccine in Healthy Adults Aged 18 Years or Older: A Randomised, Double-Blind, Placebo-Controlled, Phase 2 Trial.  *The Lancet*. 396 (10249). pp. 479–488.

F.C. Zhu et al. 2020b. Safety, Tolerability, and Immunogenicity of a Recombinant Adenovirus Type-5 Vectored COVID-19 Vaccine: A Dose-Escalation, Open-Label, Non-Randomised, First-In-Human Trial. *The Lancet*. 395. pp. 1845–1854.

F. Zhu et al. 2022a. Safety and Immunogenicity of a Live-Attenuated Influenza Virus Vector-Based Intranasal SARS-CoV-2 Vaccine in Adults: Randomised, Double-Blind, Placebo-Controlled, Phase 1 and 2 Trials. *The Lancet Respiratory Medicine*. 10. pp. 749–760.

F. Zhu et al. 2022b. Safety and Immunogenicity of a Recombinant Adenovirus Type-5-Vectored COVID-19 Vaccine with a Homologous Prime-Boost Regimen in  Healthy Participants Aged 6 Years and Above: A Randomised, Double-Blind, Placebo-Controlled, Phase 2b Trial. *Clinical Infectious Diseases: An Official Publication of the Infectious Diseases Society of America*. 75. pp. e783–e791.

www.ingramcontent.com/pod-product-compliance
Lightning Source LLC
Chambersburg PA
CBHW041837110726
48006CB00020B/2652